*To Cecilia and Vanessa*

*My prayer for your maximum healing:*

*As humanity struggles to rise up*

*From the ashes of what once was...*

*May your souls gracefully guide you*

*To an emerging light that shines*

*From a place that has always been*

*And forever will be...*

There is an increasing sense that certain ancient and esoteric healing practices, long ignored by Western Science, may in fact represent profound insights into the very nature of healing...

In western society, health is defined in strictly clinical terms by physicians. Sickness is disruption, imbalance, and the manifestation of malevolent forces in the flesh. Health and healing represent a state of balance, of harmony, and for most societies it is something holy...

— Wade Davis Ph.D.

# MaXimum Healing

*Your East-West Guide*

*to Natural Health*

## Pennyroyal Press, Inc

*Visit our web site @* MAXHEALING.com
*or call us at* 1–800–NBC–4545

Library of congress catalog card number:

ISBN: 0-9632811-2-7

Cover Design:  Joe Reynolds
Cover Photography: Robert Coletti
Text Design and layout: David Deranian, Digital Arts and Sciences.
Text Editing: Lauren Maddison
Text Chart Design: Joel Price
Text Recipes: Nancy Dunn and Connie MacSweeney

Manufactured in The United States of America

First Edition: January 1999

# ACKNOWLEDGMENTS

My Thanks To:

Nancy Dunn and Connie Gray MacSweeney for their tireless efforts and dedication, not to mention their world famous recipes.

Joel Price for Charts and Graphs.

William McAuliffe for his backup support at all times.

Joe Reynolds for his superior Cover Design efforts.

David Deranian and his Digital Arts and Sciences Layout crew.

Ken and Sam Carfagno for their Mark One Ltd. support.

Jeffrey Alan Denner esq. for his advice and support.

Thomas Tam for his special guidance with Ta'i Ch'i exercises.

Lauren Maddison for her superb edits.

Sandra Satterwhite for her publishing support.

Eric Kampmann and Gail Kump at Midpoint for their patience and faith.

## SPECIAL ACKNOWLEDGMENT

A special heartfelt thank you to Joan Wilder for her tireless labors on this book. Her literary expertise and months of hard work remain the backbone of Maximum Healing. Without her dedication, this book would have never been possible.

# Contents

PART I

CHAPTER 3

# The New Medicine:
# Blending East and West

## PART II: THE ANCIENT EAST

CHAPTER 4

# The Five Energies

CHAPTER 5

# Introduction to the Five Human Types:
# Establishing Bio-Individuality

CHAPTER 6

# What Type Are You?

CHAPTER 7  Wood

CHAPTER 11  ## Water

CHAPTER 12

## Five Simple Ta'i Ch'i Exercises

## PART III: THE MODERN WEST

CHAPTER 13

## The Modern West

CHAPTER 14

## Basic Dietary Principles for Maximum Healing

CHAPTER 17

# Fighting Cancer and Heart Disease with Food: The Magnificent Seven Phytonutrients and the Top 25 Foods

CHAPTER 16

# Supplementing the Fight Against Disease: Vitamins, Minerals, and Other Natural Medicines

CHAPTER 17

# The Spirit Ill-at-Ease

# MaXimum
# Healing

*Your East-West Guide*

*to Natural Health*

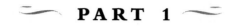

# PART 1

CHAPTER 1

# Redefining
# Health and Healing

*Beyond the world*
*of physical things*
*there is a higher, spiritual realm*
*of forms or ideas*
*beyond matter or mechanism.*

— *PLATO*

## THE SPIRIT OF HEALING

Over the past 16 years as a nutritional and wholistic therapist, I have worked with nearly 50,000 patients. With each consultation, I have become increasingly aware that nature has equipped each of us with the ability to heal. It has also become clear to me that somewhere in the extremes of modern life we have lost this ability. But just exactly what is healing and why does it seem to elude us?

I believe the answer has something to do with the quality of the lives we are living. If, for a moment, we take a break from our everyday attitudes and look deeply within, we can see beneath the surface of life to a force inside us that animates us, and lifts us up, and fills us with energy. Although we aren't often conscious of this inner aspect of our being, we unconsciously acknowledge it when we remark that a particular person is "full of life," or "has a lot of spirit." Clearly, we recognize a transcendent, spirit-like quality in other human beings, even if we don't realize it.

I believe it is just this spiritual essence that holds the key to our healing potential. Although many of us talk about spirit, the truth is that as a culture we have lost touch with it, along with our wholeness — the awareness of ourselves as spiritual, as well as, physical beings. In order to heal, we must become whole. Yet without a spiritual sense of ourselves, we are left less than whole, disassociated, and out of touch with a most integral part of ourselves. It's easy to see why this has happened. Our culture has an extremely materialistic bias which maintains that only physical things are real, while it invalidates internal realities based on feelings and beliefs. Because of this, people often respond to spirituality with misunderstanding and mistrust. A good many of us believe that spirituality can only be found in religious institutions, or that it is something mystical or mysterious.

But spirituality is simpler than all that, as much a part of daily life as the air we breath. Spirituality is all around us everyday. It is the Divine inspiration we feel at the birth of a child, the joy that moves us with the coming of Spring, or the grief we feel at the death of a loved one. Spirituality is reflected in the unique, unseen energetic quality of each and every human being. Spirit is everything that is not material: unseen life-force, dreams, hopes, beliefs, emotions.

Intuition, too, is a type of internal, spiritual phenomenon that science can't measure and our culture doesn't value. Consequently, we don't trust ourselves or what we know in our hearts to be true. This results in a separation between the mind and the heart. We may even say we care about soulful and spiritual phenomena, but often the bottom line is that we don't believe that things we can't see can affect us. This separation between our hearts and minds – the denial of our spiritual natures – creates a terrible rift in the fabric of our beings that has resulted in a grievous lack of self-integration and self-esteem in a vast cross-section of Americans. But how can we possibly find the key to loving ourselves if we are disconnected from our true nature?

Herbert Maslow, the esteemed human behaviorist, taught that the greatest of all human needs is self-esteem. Greater than our need for food, shelter, or clothing is our need to establish a "true self identity." Without this, we cannot determine our values, our priorities or our reason for living. Yet, to love, to be whole, and to heal we must know and be *who we are*. The truth is that who we are is not just our material bodies, but *also* souls and spirits and minds. Not everything can be measured by science; not everything can be known or understood or treated from the outside. Human beings are a miraculous complex of physical (material) and non-physical (spiritual) energy systems. Like the electricity that causes a light bulb to become illuminated, we, too, are powered by an unseen life-force.

To maximize our true healing potential, we need to begin by acknowledging this unseen power as it expresses itself in the subtle energies of our minds, spirits, and souls. These parts of ourselves — our beliefs, intuitions, thoughts, feelings — must be cared for with as much attention as we devote to our physical, visible bodies. We need to acknowledge that the body, mind, spirit, and soul are connected *in a practical sense*. We cannot hate or resent our boss and pretend that those feelings have nothing to do with our hypertension and indigestion. We can't keep a stiff upper lip when our hearts are heavy, refusing to express our grief; eventually the grief will find physical expression. Emotions are real and have the power to affect the workings of the body.

For the purposes of this work, I use the word *mind* to

refer to the whole spectrum of unseen life-force — the spiritual phenomena which include emotions, intuition, thoughts, beliefs, and feelings. Perhaps, as we become more tuned-in to these internal dynamics, we will come to distinguish between them more clearly. For now, it is enough to acknowledge their presence, their power, and the mysterious and wondrous aspect of life they represent. Without this acknowledgment we can never be whole and we cannot heal.

## THE SPIRIT OF WHOLISM

Just as we need to claim our wholeness and right relationship with ourselves as physical, mental, and spiritual beings, we also need to claim our rightful place in the world as a unique part of a greater whole. This awareness is all but lost in modern technological life. Once our ancestors lived in tune with Nature. They knew who they were because they recognized their intimate relationship to the big, consistent cycles that brought seed in Spring, growth in Summer, bounty in Fall. We Westerners, however, live as though we can conquer and dominate Nature with no detrimental effects. Our technological prowess has led us to believe that we are in no way dependent upon or connected with the great cycles of birth and growth by which our ancestors lived and died. But we *are* part of Nature, and Nature lives within us. We cannot prosper and remain separate from the natural world, for to do so is to remain severed from our own true natures. If we are to claim our power to heal, we must reclaim our awareness of 'whole-ism.' As these fundamental changes in awareness filter down through our lives, we begin to change the way we think. As we become whole, we will begin to question many of our previous assumptions.

*Just as we need to claim our wholeness and right
relationship with ourselves as physical, mental, and spiritual
beings, we also need to claim our rightful place in the world
as a unique part of a greater whole.*

Another result of living in a materialistic, externally-focused culture is that we have lost our belief that we can affect our own healing. Instead, we think that only an external agent, a doctor in most cases, can fix us when we're sick. Yet study after study, as well as the many personal histories being published today, show that people who take an active role in their own health care protocols tend to have far more positive results than those who don't. Again, the problem involves changing the beliefs which denigrate our subtle energy by denigrating our own experiences, feelings, and intuitions.

This disinclination to trust our own healing instincts has been fostered by a mechanically-biased culture and its medical philosophy which denies that any kind of spiritual life-force energy can have an effect on our health. And, while some of us may believe our emotions wield some power in our everyday lives, it's likely that we still don't understand how they can influence healing. To most of us, an inflammation remains an inflammation; a cyst is a cyst.

Just as we must acknowledge our need to be good stewards of our physical life-force, we cannot ignore the effect of our emotional life on our health. We can't expect to be healthy in body, mind, and spirit if we don't pay attention to each of them. We must give our bodies good fuel and regular exercise. We maintain our mental health by exercising (in other words, acknowledging and releasing) our emotions, and by stimulating our minds. We nurture our spirits with music, meditation, or spiritual practice. However we choose to live our lives, we cannot remind ourselves often enough that these three elements — body, mind, and spirit — are inseparable elements of the *whole* human being.

One of my patients, a man in his 60's, came to see me after being diagnosed with a rare form of cancer. His doctors had told him that he had three months to live. Ed, as I will call him, had had a lifetime of crippling fear. He was afraid of many things, but at the top of the list was flying. At the time of his diagnosis, Ed's daughter was due to graduate from UCLA in four months' time and he dearly wanted to be present. A few weeks later, he decided that he was not only going to live long enough to congratulate his daughter on her graduation, but that he was going to get on an airplane for the first time in his life and fly to California. Feeling as though he no longer had anything to lose, Ed bought a round-trip ticket. Challenging his most crippling fear, he flew to Los Angeles for her graduation. Shortly after his return — about five months after the doctors had given him his 3-month death sentence — Ed's doctors found that his cancer had gone into full remission. Now, some eight years later, he remains healthy and cancer-free.

Everything we do (how we deal with stress, what we think, feel, and believe, how we choose and prepare the food we eat, the kinds of medicines we take) creates an energetic response that either enhances or diminishes our life-force energy. We must recognize that all parts of ourselves, whether flesh, feeling, or faith are different conduits for the same single animating life force.

## VITALISTIC AND MECHANISTIC BELIEF SYSTEMS

What humankind knows and believes about healing and wellness has changed continually from the beginning of time.

Our healing systems also differ vastly from one culture to another. Although we have been steeped in the modern material world view, luckily we have another model with which to inform our changing ideas. To glimpse such a model, we can look both to our own past and to the healing systems of Eastern cultures, most notably ancient Chinese Medicine, which has been my dominant influence. This system of thought is rooted in a belief that all life is endowed with a special vitalizing life-force which both animates matter and forms it. In this system, human beings are seen to be part of the natural world and subject to its laws. *Vitalism*, as this belief system is called, holds that although man participates in the process, *it is Nature that ultimately heals*. Health, then, is a matter of complying with Nature so as to most beneficially cultivate the life-force that flows through us.

Perhaps you can remember your grandparents or the woman up the street or the old family doctor as vitalists. When you were sick they would have wanted to know what was going on at school, how you were feeling, whether you'd gotten a chill at recess. They might have questioned you about what you'd eaten for breakfast, whether you'd been properly dressed for the weather, what was happening at home before you left for school. They understood, innately, that human beings were whole mind-body systems comprised of subtle interwoven energies which profoundly affected health. They ministered to your feelings and questioned you about your interaction with your world. They knew that good health was the result of adapting to the dictates of Nature — both inside and out.

On the other hand, modern materialistic philosophy can be described as a mechanistic system. Mechanism is distinguished by its belief that people are separate from Nature and, like machines, can be analyzed and treated in isolation from the greater whole. Just as mechanism separates people from nature, it separates the human mind and spirit from the body.

Although mechanistic philosophy (which formed the basis of the Western scientific medical model) still dominates our thinking, modern science continues to move beyond it. The advanced study of physics has established that all of life can be reduced to a common element billions of times smaller than an atom. Quanta, as they are called by physicists, are neither matter nor energy, but a kind of basic essence from which both are formed. When reduced to its smallest parts, then, the entire phenomenal world is comprised of the same basic "stuff." Put another way, the science of sub-atomic physics has established that we are not separate from each other or from Nature, but connected in one vast energetic field. This is quantum field theory and it is a first cousin to vitalism. Science, then, has proven what the ancients intuitively knew to be true. This mechanistic validation of vitalistic principles is but a greater validation of whole-ism.

*We are not separate from each other or from Nature,*
*but connected in one vast energetic field.*

In the past 25 years or so, bolstered by the success of science in "proving" what had always been essentially intuitive knowledge, our Western world has begun to reclaim a more vitalistic model of living and healing. Many techniques from vitalistic medicinal systems have begun to filter into our everyday world, and alternative therapies and complementary medicine are becoming more and more common. Today, there are many programs at respected medical centers which use a variety of preventative techniques to treat illnesses. Nutritional therapy as well as mind-body medicine (which includes such stress reduction techniques as meditation, breathing, Yoga and Tai Ch'i exercises) have proven themselves effective in treating a vast array of medical problems. A host of double-blind studies — the only way we Westerners will really believe something is true — illustrate how cultivation and manipulation of the subtle life-force heal disease and create vibrant health.

A recent study of Finnish men indicated that those who didn't feel love or hope were 20% more likely to die of cancer than those men who did. Equally fascinating is the research being done at the Institute of Heartmath, a think-tank in Santa Cruz, California. Researchers there are monitoring changes in the bodies of subjects as they practice simple exercises that focus loving feelings in the heart. Not only does the actual heart beat change in a matter of minutes, but these changes dramatically raise the body's levels of anti-aging hormones, strengthen several chemical indicators of immune system function, balance the sympathetic and parasympathetic nervous systems, and lower a hormone that promotes aging and illness.

Every day the evidence is mounting to prove that a subtle life-force profoundly affects the course of the physical body. We are coming to experience what the ancient Chinese knew 5,000 years ago — health and illness are not random events, but largely the result of how naturally we cultivate our life-force. Of course, knowledge is one thing; incorporating it into our lives is another. Experience brings belief, and belief calls for more experience. In order to begin to harness our true healing power, we need to change our minds about how we view who we are and what we believe. Perhaps looking at the world through the eyes of a higher consciousness can be our greatest healing experience.

One of my patient's stories is particularly vivid in my

mind — I will call her Kathy. At the time that I worked with her, she was a young woman in her early 30s. For the past several years she'd suffered from extreme food sensitivities. There were very few foods she could tolerate without getting sick. She became so congested when she ate dairy, wheat, and yeast that she couldn't function. She also had a number of immunological problems. I muscle tested her and weaned her from the foods to which she showed sensitivity. Kathy came to the office frequently — once a week for the first month, then every two or three weeks.

During the four months I worked with Kathy, we got to know each other better. Eventually, she told me that she'd been living with her fiancee for ten years and wanted to get married, but he didn't. She never mentioned it, though, for fear of losing him. As time passed, she began to feel increasingly bothered by the fact that she wasn't telling him how she felt. We talked about this, and I gently urged her to stand up for herself, her needs, and her feelings. I stressed that I thought it was important for her to express herself. Eventually, she mustered up the conviction and confronted him. Though he remained unmoved by this honest expression of her needs, she stood her ground and a short while later they split up. Although Kathy was initially upset by the turn of events, almost immediately all of her food sensitivities disappeared! When we met in the weeks following the break-up she was sad, but she felt free from the fear that had bound her for years. She had liberated her heart, and her heart had liberated her body of its debilitating symptoms.

Our life-force resides in our hearts, in our cells, in our thoughts and beliefs. Whether your heart hurts from sadness and grief or from blocked arteries, it is all blocked energy. Natural healing involves cultivating and enhancing all your life-force, whether it's through the kinds of medicines you use, the foods you eat, what you think, how you act, or what you believe.

---

*Health and illness are not random events, but largely the result of how naturally we cultivate our life-force.*

## PUTTING IT ALL TOGETHER: THE MIND-BODY

In energetic terms, then, there is no difference between the mind and the body. When a client comes to me with an ailment, it is necessary to look at all the influences that affect the problem. Indirectly, this means we look at the entire mind-body environment, since everything is related to everything in a whole system. It is my thesis that only by blending the best of Western, mechanistic and chemical knowledge with the best of the ancient vitalistic Chinese approach, can we become whole beings and claim our maximum healing potential.

# CHAPTER 2

# The Power to Heal

*From Wonder*
*into Wonder*
*Existence Opens*

— *LAO TZU*

Coinciding with my 20 years of formal education, research, and practice in the science of nutrition, I have been a student of the art of Chinese Medicine. Although nutritional therapy represents the primary focus of my life's work, my understanding and practice of Chinese Medicine have dramatically changed the way I work. I was once more adamant in my belief that nourishing the body with the proper foods was the only way to good health, but I have since realized that nourishing the mind is equally important. Regardless of a client's illness, in most cases, I now believe their disharmonies need to be addressed on the mental-emotional level before they can be addressed on the physical. In order for healing to take place, the patient must first be viewed as whole.

Chinese Medicine was one of the first formalized medical systems — along with Ayurvedic — to have established healing protocols that were mind-body oriented. Thus inspired and influenced by the Chinese approach to healing, my work has expanded beyond one-dimensional nutritional therapy and now includes a more integrative, wholistic approach.

It is important to note here that ancient Chinese Medicine has never been extremely standardized. Rather, it is an artful science that has been customized by each person who practices it. The knowledge has been passed down through the generations from family to family, each altering and adding to it. My understanding and application of Chinese medicinal principles is very much in keeping with this. I have developed a hybrid of ancient Chinese healing arts and modern techniques in all of the therapies I use. In my dietary work, for instance, I blend the latest in nutritional, chemical knowledge with the Chinese approach, a personalized system based on the energetic properties of food, something I will discuss in more detail later in the book.

Chinese Medicine encompasses eight healing arts, known today as the Eight Strands of the Brocade. These eight, which have been passed from family to family over centuries, make up the primary pillars of Chinese Medicine. Each one is a model of energy healing. These classical forms include the following: nutrition; herbal therapy (natural medicines); occlusion (mind–body medicine); contact thermogenesis (energy healing); acupressure; acupuncture; diagnosis; and massage. I work with four of the eight, and this book will focus on the following three: nutritional therapy; mind–body medicine; and natural medicine (which today includes vitamins and minerals). Before delving into these basic therapeutic approaches, let's take a closer look at the fundamental belief systems of Chinese Medicine.

## SIMPLIFIED FUNDAMENTALS OF CHINESE MEDICINE

The ancient Chinese belief system begins with the idea that all of life exists within the web of Nature. In this context, all things are seen to be interconnected and interdependent. Events influence all parts within a whole concurrently: what is good for one part is good for all because everything and everyone is part of the same whole. This way of thinking is reflected in the ancient Chinese approach to health and healing, which sees symptoms in relationship to the whole mind-body, and sees human beings in relationship to all of Nature. In this thought system, good health is seen to be the result of healthy interactions among all parts and systems of the mind-body.

Allopathic (Western) medicine, on the other hand, targets specific sets of symptoms and treats them as though they existed in isolation from the rest of the mind-body. Often, however, medications have side-effects. They may have an impact on bodily processes and functions other than the one they are targeting. Clearly, symptoms cannot be treated as though one part of the mind-body doesn't affect another. Additionally, medicines frequently mask superficial symptoms, thereby producing a false sense of wellness. When this happens, rather than making lifestyle or dietary changes, the person does nothing and thinks she is cured. In this case, the problem that the illness reflected can take hold of the person on an even deeper level because the needs of the mind-body haven't been addressed or fulfilled, just masked. From the Chinese point of view, symptoms are seen as messages that communicate important information about what the mind-body needs.

## A PATIENT'S STORY

The following story is a first-person account in the patient's own words.

*"I was diagnosed with MS about six years ago. After two-and-a-half years of playing around with Western medicine, I didn't know what to do. I'd never been sick before in my life and I was stuck with multiple sclerosis. Thank God I'm such a die-hard optimist because it was such a dead end. Every three months I'd end up in the hospital for 10 days of steroids. Then I'd get sent home and I'd feel sicker than when I went in; it was the side-effects. After a while I realized that the side-effects of the drugs were killing me.*

*At one point, someone said to me, why don't you look for a wholistic medicine man. So I asked around and I kept hearing the name, Mark Mincolla. One day, after I'd left a message at his office, but hadn't heard back from him yet, I was in the natural food store and who should come in but Mark Mincolla and his wife! So I started going to him.*

*Mark took my history; he's wholistic medicine, so he has to know the whole story—when I got sick, how I got sick, what was going on in my life. I was very stressed at work and I was a very career-minded person. Every month I went to see Mark. Right away he changed my diet. He felt he could put out the fire in my legs, and he did. Then I started getting bladder infections, and the doctors put me on antibiotics. I couldn't break that cycle of antibiotic dependency, until finally, with Mark's diet and therapies, the antibiotic-induced infections finally went away.*

*I continue to follow the diet he put me on — low-fat, mostly vegetables and proteins. He also has me on supplements. Sometimes I cheat with food a little bit — I take my 10% leeway he allows me — but I'm feeling better to the point where, as of this past January, I went back to work. I was overwhelmed with enthusiasm to be working again. Mark has helped me to temper my enthusiasm and follow a different route to a long-lasting career. Now, I firmly let my limits be known and speak my mind when something is bothering me. I've learned how to say 'no' when it's appropriate and I work at my own pace, based on what I'm feeling and not on what I think everyone else expects of me.*

*It is great to be able to play the game of life once again and not have to watch from the sidelines. I am happy Mark is the 'manager' of my team! He helped me understand that I needed to change the rules a bit to make the game both enjoyable and winnable. It's a small miracle, really."*

Throughout the course of our work together, this patient clearly learned that all the events of her life profoundly influenced her mind and her body. I have never seen anyone work harder at respecting and positively reprogramming her subtle mind-body energies.

### CH'I

Perhaps the most fundamental concept of Chinese Medicine is the idea that all nature is powered by a subtle, invisible energy. Ch'i, as it is called, has no English translation; we don't think about invisible energy and we have no word for it. But Ch'i is just that — an unseen energetic life-force. All events and things are empowered by Ch'i and are made of Ch'i. It represents form *and* process, matter *and* energy. Ch'i is the wind that blows and the trees that bend. It is the rising of the sap and the forming of chlorophyll. Ch'i is the instinct that sends the salmon upstream to lay its eggs. It is apparent in gravity, magnetism, and electricity. Ch'i is the life that moves us, the flesh that is us. The first law of Chinese Medicine states that Ch'i *is* ever-present and everywhere.

Coupled with this is the second law of Chinese Medicine that postulates that Ch'i (unseen life-force) is in constant motion. Never stopping, it is the nature of Ch'i to continuously cycle between polar and complementary opposites: cold and hot, Winter and Summer, beginning and end, Yin and Yang. This constant movement represents all potential energy patterns, movements, and expressions in nature. When Ch'i is balanced and centered, life is in harmony.

Since the natural state of Ch'i is movement, it follows that something is wrong when movement becomes blocked. We can see examples of this in both the mind and the body. Whether cholesterol blocks circulation or repression blocks the flow of a particular emotion, both result in disease. The third law states just this. When Ch'i is blocked, there is disharmony. Translated into a healing context, we can say that when Ch'i, or energy, is out of balance, or blocked, disease results.

## DISEASE AS MESSENGER

Just as health is the natural result of a balanced condition in the body, so, too, is illness the natural result of an imbalance. Illnesses, then, are messengers indicating that the mind-body needs something. If we ignore what these messengers are communicating, increasingly serious illnesses will result. From Chinese Medicine we learn that imbalances or problems travel from one organ system to another if they are left uncorrected. What begins as a simple illness able to be treated quite easily can become a serious illness. Mildly troubling symptoms can turn into chronic and acute illness if the original problem is left untreated.

Western medicine would have us believe that we either have a disease or we don't. Most often, though, diseases develop over time when unfavorable conditions remain untreated. Chronic energy swings after too much sugar, for example, will inevitably develop into disease as time passes. I have often heard people blame the medical establishment for not correctly diagnosing them with a chronic condition without understanding that they hadn't yet developed the full range of symptoms recognizable as the particular disease. In these cases, the person has ignored how they've felt for years and failed to make dietary or lifestyle changes that would have alleviated their symptoms and reversed their progression toward a disease. Having failed to heed these messages, they eventually develop a serious illness. The mind-body first attempts to communicate to us in symptomatic whispers. If we fail to listen, however, it will scream and shout. Self-care and learning to listen to our bodies are fundamental to maximizing our health and healing potential. We must learn to recognize and respond to the body's subtlest communications.

## HEALING IS A NATURAL STATE

It is natural for Ch'i to be life-giving, just as it is natural that our bodies heal. The minute we cut ourselves, the wound begins to heal. Immediately, thousands of processes mobilize to start their healing work. All of Nature is endowed with this self-regulating spirit of renewal. Even the Earth is seen as a single entity with these abilities. The Gaia Hypothesis, set forth by British Scientist James Lovelock, postulates that the Earth is a living being that can mobilize a multitude of processes to counteract the changing influences to which it is continually subject. This allows our planet to maintain its equilibrium, despite the natural changes to which she must continually adapt. This reflects the fundamental Chinese philosophy that an organism's ability to adapt to changing conditions is the single most important measure of its good health.

In the crush of technology and the external focus that has characterized our recent culture, most of us Westerners have lost our sense of being connected to Nature. We are part of the Earth, though, and the same forces that operate in Nature, operate in us. Each one of us is a microcosm — or smaller version — of the Earth as a whole. We are part of the Earth just as the Earth is part of the universe. These patterns in Nature reveal the underlying connection that we have with the universe. Existence is revealed to us as a set of carved Chinese boxes, each one nestled inside the next. We have stars, comets and planets within the universe; humanity, seas, and fire within the Earth; blood, mind, and spirit within humanity; electrons, protons, and nuclei within atoms. Our experience and the world is comprised of a vast and never-ending whole of interconnected parts that each have corresponding cycles, processes, and tendencies. And just as the sailor learns to navigate the currents of wind and water to his best advantage, we must recognize ourselves as part of the natural world and learn to adapt to its dictates.

On the most basic level, we innately understand natural law. For instance, if we eat nothing, eventually we will die; if we eat too much, we gain weight. If we try to stay awake, we will eventually fall asleep; if we try too hard to sleep, we will stay awake. There are much more subtle laws, however, and Chinese medicine contains a wealth of wisdom about them. Their medicine is the result of thousands of years of observing nature and detailing its ways. To know the ways of Nature is to know how to balance, cultivate and, consequently, enhance our life-force (Ch'i). The Chinese have classified many characteristics of Ch'i. The following section contains a very brief overview that will spark your innate understanding of the energy that continuously flows through you.

## YIN AND YANG
## AND THE FIVE ENERGIES

In Chinese thought, all of Nature is seen to arise from a single unified oneness. From this oneness, referred to as the Tao (God), comes all being which is differentiated from the oneness by the very fact that it has a separate identity. Beingness, by which I mean everything that can be spoken of and named, is made up of opposites: night and day, tall and short, full and empty, internal and external, cold and hot. These complementary poles both form and define all things; it is impossible to know light without darkness, front without back, hot without cold, sorrow without joy. These archetypal extremes are symbolically referred to as Yin and Yang.

Although Yin and Yang are opposites, they are complementary parts of a single whole that balance each other. These symbolic, complementary opposites are constantly interweaving, as day gives way to night, up to down, movement to stillness. One aspect is continually changing into another. Yin is constantly changing into Yang, and Yang is constantly changing into Yin. After the pendulum swings to its most extreme point, it falls in the other direction. In this light, we understand the saying that the darkest hour is just before dawn.

While the Chinese use Yin and Yang to describe the cyclical nature of the world through complementary opposites, they further divide the world into Five Energies. Just as the seasons flow from one to the other, Wood, Fire, Earth, Metal and Water are used to organize and understand the underlying energy movement and cyclical development of all things, from beginning to end and back again. The Five Energies have a variety of corresponding aspects to them that can be applied to people, places, foods, herbs, processes, and ideas.

## THE FIVE ENERGIES

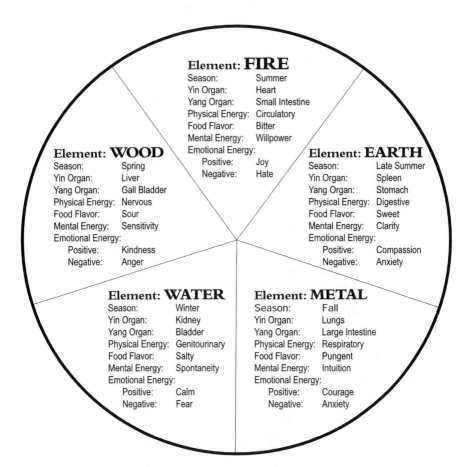

**Element: FIRE**
| Season: | Summer |
| Yin Organ: | Heart |
| Yang Organ: | Small Intestine |
| Physical Energy: | Circulatory |
| Food Flavor: | Bitter |
| Mental Energy: | Willpower |
| Emotional Energy: | |
| Positive: | Joy |
| Negative: | Hate |

**Element: WOOD**
| Season: | Spring |
| Yin Organ: | Liver |
| Yang Organ: | Gall Bladder |
| Physical Energy: | Nervous |
| Food Flavor: | Sour |
| Mental Energy: | Sensitivity |
| Emotional Energy: | |
| Positive: | Kindness |
| Negative: | Anger |

**Element: EARTH**
| Season: | Late Summer |
| Yin Organ: | Spleen |
| Yang Organ: | Stomach |
| Physical Energy: | Digestive |
| Food Flavor: | Sweet |
| Mental Energy: | Clarity |
| Emotional Energy: | |
| Positive: | Compassion |
| Negative: | Anxiety |

**Element: WATER**
| Season: | Winter |
| Yin Organ: | Kidney |
| Yang Organ: | Bladder |
| Physical Energy: | Genitourinary |
| Food Flavor: | Salty |
| Mental Energy: | Spontaneity |
| Emotional Energy: | |
| Positive: | Calm |
| Negative: | Fear |

**Element: METAL**
| Season: | Fall |
| Yin Organ: | Lungs |
| Yang Organ: | Large Intestine |
| Physical Energy: | Respiratory |
| Food Flavor: | Pungent |
| Mental Energy: | Intuition |
| Emotional Energy: | |
| Positive: | Courage |
| Negative: | Anxiety |

I use the Five Energies as a tool for personalizing nutritional therapy by matching The Five Constitutional Types with the corresponding Food Flavors that maximize their healing potential. We will present this system in later chapters.

## THE WAYS OF ENERGY: HOW POWER MOVES

Just as Earth experiences the forces of Nature, so, too, do human beings. Ch'i, which encompasses these forces, is seen to be in constant movement — cycling from one pole to the other in a continuous ebb and flow. By understanding the nature of Ch'i we can facilitate its unfettered movement. In keeping with this, the Chinese classified many forms, characteristics, attributes, and movements of Ch'i so as to be able to manipulate and balance their vital life-force.

## THE FOUR SOURCES OF CH'I*

In this system, Ch'i is understood to be derived from four sources. They are as follows.

The process of respiration receives Ch'i from oxygen.
The process of digestion receives Ch'i from food.
The process of circulation receives Ch'i from the blood.
The process of excretion receives Ch'i from detoxification.

The above examples help us Westerners to better understand the practical aspects of Ch'i. Oxygen, for instance, is appreciated by both East and West as the most vital source of all life-giving power. It is easy for us to grasp the role it plays in health and healing. Science tells us that as much as 75% of the human body is comprised of water, and 90% of water is comprised of oxygen. When the body receives the correct amount of oxygen, it is able to create carbon dioxide in the proper ratios, forming a gas which the body can eliminate. This process of oxidation allows the body to maintain a normal temperature which fortifies the immune capabilities of the glands and organs. On the other hand, if oxygen is not sufficiently supplied to the bloodstream, carbon monoxide is formed, which is not readily eliminated from the body, thus upsetting the maintenance of normal body temperatures. This situation allows a multitude of environmental stresses to invade the glands and organs, setting the stage for disease.

Just like oxygen, food (through digestion) is also a primary carrier of Ch'i. Although Western medicine has yet to work with nutrition medicinally, the Chinese classified it as one of their healing modalities as well as one of the primary sources of Ch'i.

## THE SIX MANIFESTATIONS OF CH'I*

When Ch'i moves, it manifests in some form or another. Chinese theory tells of six manifestations of naturally-directed Ch'i.

> When Ch'i congeals, it creates matter.
> When Ch'i disperses, it creates space.
> When Ch'i animates, it creates life.
> When Ch'i flows, it creates health.
> When Ch'i is blocked, it creates sickness.
> When Ch'i departs, it creates death.

In the true spirit of Chinese medicine, the primary focus of my work is to enhance the flowing manifestation of Ch'i, while avoiding the blockage of Ch'i.

When Ch'i flows there is health; when Ch'i is blocked, there is disease. The previously mentioned example of cholesterol blockages can, in most cases, be treated successfully with diet and/or natural medicines; reducing the intake of saturated fat rids the arteries of plaque deposits and allows the blood to flow freely. Fish oils, lecithin, and niacin (vitamin B3) aid in this process. In some cases, natural medicines, such as these, along with dietary modifications, are all that is necessary to reverse the condition.

---

* My understanding of the Four Sources and the Six Manifestations of Ch'i were taught to me by Master Ni, Hua-Ching.

*When Ch'i flows, there is health;*
*when Ch'i is blocked, there is disease.*

To relieve other ailments, however, problems need to be addressed on both the seen and unseen levels. In such cases, it isn't only physical reasons that prevent an organ or bodily system from maintaining a balanced wellness. Often, there are unresolved emotional issues that further block the flow of Ch'i to the point of dysfunction. The Chinese Five Emotions theory is very instructive in this area. It postulates that emotional energy is a real force which must be released and expressed. If it isn't released externally, it will be stored in the body. In Chapters 7–11 we will explore this system with its specific correspondences between emotions and organ systems.

Just as the heart becomes diseased from a blockage of Ch'i-giving blood, the lungs become diseased if they are blocked from receiving oxygen through a breakdown in the process of respiration. Asthma is an ailment which we in the West commonly link to both emotional and physical blockages. This parallels the Chinese belief that unexpressed grief stores in the lungs if not properly expressed. In this case, mind-body protocols such as meditation and prayer must be employed to ensure recovery.

Frequently, diet is also a contributing factor. I've had hundreds of patients whose asthma has been relieved by restricting or eliminating dairy. Dairy products create phlegm and mucus which often block the lungs, obstructing respiration. Again, we have to look at the whole individual to see what factors are at work.

Our goal remains to find ways to facilitate the movement of Ch'i, or energy, within the body. Nutrition is a wonderful tool for this.

Taking the example of digestion and assimilation, there are many people with an inability to break down calcium because of inadequate hydrochloric (digestive) acids in the stomach. When the body cannot break down calcium it must be stored someplace, frequently as kidney stones or arterial blockages, so this is a serious (and common) problem.

Interestingly, stress is often the first culprit. When the body is stressed, the adrenal glands chemically stress the thyroid gland, causing it to stop producing calcitonin, a calcium digestive hormone. This cycle can initiate an array of problems, since digestion is vital for unlocking nutrients from the foods that contain them.

So often, we can work backwards from symptoms to find where the body's natural processes were blocked from doing their job. In many cases, allopathic medicines mask the real problem, causing the body to become more and more out of balance, setting the stage for more complex levels of dysfunction.

In the next chapter I will give a more thorough overview of the three healing brocades which I deal with in this book: nutritional therapy, natural medicines, and mind-body medicine. I believe that these three approaches can be used as the core conduits of Ch'i to maximize your healing potential.

# CHAPTER 3

# The New Medicine:
# Blending East and West

In many ways, Western medicine and ancient Chinese medicine are opposites. Yet, as the cultural gap between them narrows, we see how well they work together. Their mutual compatibility exemplifies the well-known concept of Yin and Yang. On the simplest level, Yin and Yang are symbols for any two polar opposites that comprise a single whole; Eastern and Western medicine represent two sides of the same coin.

As our culture becomes more global, our view of the world changes. Where we once identified only with the people and places closest to us, we now identify with the wider world as part of ourselves. In the same way, Eastern and Western medicines, previously worlds apart, are beginning to come together. I remember the 1950's as a time when West was West and East was East. No one had ever heard of stress or any number of other mind-body approaches to healing. Now, stress management is known to be as critical to heart health as any cholesterol medication. Although the old medical model still has a very strong foothold, things are changing, and a new hybrid medicine is emerging that blends the best of the Eastern and Western systems.

## PREVENTION

In my practice we employ both systems, taking the best from each. It continues to amaze me how well the Eastern and Western models combine to create a much more complete healing system than either one alone. The most important contribution Eastern medicine has made to the Western way of thinking is its focus on prevention. Prevention involves supporting and enhancing the body's own natural healing system as the first line of defense against disease. As sensible and simple as this approach is, it has only in the past few years attracted the attention of Western medicine, which is predominantly disease-oriented and applied only after illness has already occurred. But why not keep illness from happening in the first place? We've all heard the old maxim that an ounce of prevention is worth a pound of cure. It really is much easier and much simpler to make a consistent effort at being healthy than to fight disease.

Just as efficiency experts emulate the habits of successful entrepreneurs, our medical researchers would do well to study the habits of healthy people and learn from them. It is astounding to me how many research dollars have gone into devising ways to attack disease, while little effort is expended in learning how to prevent it. It's as if we've spent all our time studying the habits of the enemy rather than reinforcing the walls of our own precious immune fortress. We've become so accustomed to thinking about health care as disease-oriented rather than wellness-oriented, it's hard for many of us to take prevention seriously. But all that is changing.

## THE AMAZING HEALING SYSTEM

The goal of prevention is to fortify the body's natural ability to fend off disease before it has a chance to take hold. This approach has grown out of the awareness that healing is a natural function of the body. Not only do we have an amazing immune system defending the body against ever-present viruses, cancers, and bacteria, but the body is engaged in an on-going process of self-repair. From the unseen realms to the most obvious cuts and breaks, the body's intelligence is at work.

The immune system, comprised of trillions of specialized cells, has three main types of T-cells (immune cells). One group, the Killer T-cells, constantly patrols the body searching out foreign invaders. When a Killer T-cell encounters a virus, tumor, bacteria or other micro-enemy, it communicates this information to another group of cells called Helper T-cells, which have several strategies for destroying a foreign body. After these 'Pacman'-like cells destroy the invader's walls, they surround the enemy with their spider-like tentacles and release enzymes that dismantle the cell's component parts. These remarkable cells then study the dead invader and transmit chemical alarms throughout the body that teach other immune cells how to recognize and remember the invaders. These specialized "memory" cells then remember the invader's characteristics for the rest of the person's life. If the memory cells encounter the invader again, even years later, they are able to recognize it very quickly and can alert the Killer T-cells immediately.  After this cellular search and destroy mission is completed, another group called Suppressor T-cells arrive to call off the fight and clean up the debris.

Our bodies continually host a multitude of foreign invaders including cancer cells, bacteria, viruses, fungi and various allergens capable of creating disease at all times. Only a healthy and vigorous immune system is able to resist their advance. Clearly, diet and natural medicines directly affect the production and potency of immune cells, the majority of which are white blood cells. This is why it is so important to nourish and enhance all the components of the immune system. And, since all bodily systems are connected to each other (like the old song about the hip bone being connected to the thigh bone), whatever is good for any one part or system of the body ultimately enhances the working of the immune system.

The primary components of the immune system include the thymus gland, which produces tens of millions of T-cells every minute. The bone marrow, too, produces millions of white blood cells that act as primary immune cells, while the spleen, the lymph nodes and the ducts produce a variety of proteins and chemical messengers, such as interferon, which kill invaders including ever-present cancer cells. As we can see, no matter what therapies, drugs, or surgery a person may use to cure a disease, when all is said and done, it is the body's own healing system that does the work.

When disease has taken a very strong hold, clearly the body's healing and immune systems have been overwhelmed and disabled. Invasive therapies, then, work by destroying enough of the diseased parts to allow the healing system to cope with the rest and to come back on-line. The tricky part of using invasive therapies is that they can and frequently do destroy the very cells, tissues, and organs of the immune system that are so critically important for healing.

Many studies today illustrate just how well nutritional support can protect the immune system while a body undergoes chemotherapy, radiation, or antibiotics. Remember, these therapies are not smart bombs; they don't only target the cancer or infected cells, but the healthy cells as well. Antibiotics, for instance, kill off a large population of the body's good bacteria along with the invasive ones. That's why it is important to eat acidophilus and other active bacterial cultures (found in yogurt) when taking antibiotics.

Studies indicate that vitamins C, E and other antioxidants can protect vital immune organs, while also enhancing tumor reduction, in cancer patients undergoing radiation treatments. Vitamin E also protects the heart from damage caused by adriamycin, a chemotherapy drug, and seems to have an anti-cancer component as well. These antioxidant nutrients are abundantly found in fresh fruits and vegetables, especially those with the darkest colors. (Please see Chapter 15 for detailed information on the antioxidants in foods.) Many other studies, including those performed by the Nobel prize-winning Linus Pauling (whose Nobel prize was awarded for his research on Vitamin C) indicate that cancer patients who undergo nutritional support live longer and do better than those who do not.

It is even more effective, however, to support our precious immune systems and enhance our life-force with good nutrition, natural medicine, and mind–body behavior techniques *before* we get sick. The following section gives an overview of these basic immune enhancing approaches, which comprise the bulk of this book. It begins with a look at the Standard American Diet (S.A.D.).

## A PATIENT'S STORY

(The following story is a first-person account in the patient's own words.)

*"For two or three years before going to Mark, I'd been having severe abdominal pain. I couldn't sleep at night, all of that. The doctors were telling me it was this one thing — I can't remember what it was called. I was trying to live with it… you put up with what you have to… until I started bleeding from the bowel and ended up in the*

hospital. When I left, my doctor told me that I had to have an extensive operation, even though they weren't sure it would be successful. I didn't know what to do.

Meanwhile, my daughter had been going to Mark and had been trying to get me to go. Pain's a great motivator, so finally I went to see him. I was really in tough shape. I had very high blood pressure and the bowel problem, and I'd already had cancer, so I didn't need anything else. I didn't know how he was going to help me, but I went.

Right away he changed my diet extensively. It seemed that all the things I was told to use when I left the hospital were absolutely the opposite of what I could tolerate. I couldn't take regular bread or any milk products — I still can't take them — though I can have one type of bread: sourdough rice bread. My basic diet now is low-fat proteins like chicken, and various combinations of high-starch and low-starch vegetables mostly. And he put me on various supplements and the pain went, finally. It took a little while but it went away. It's gone.

So, I'm on a strict diet and I follow it, but it's been a year and my pain is gone. I feel so good. Can you believe it? I'm so grateful to him, I owe him my life. Also, I was on two blood pressure pills a day because my blood pressure was so high — I'd already had a stroke — but after I'd been going to Mark for about six months, my doctor lowered it from two pills to one. My husband says my blood pressure is like a kid's!

I see Mark about every 6 to 8 weeks. When I went to see my doctor afterwards, he was a little concerned because I'd lost weight, but of course I wasn't eating any sweets or anything since going to Mark. But when I explained to him I was out of pain he said, 'Look, anything that works that well, just keep doing that.' And that's what I do."

## THE S.A.D.
## (STANDARD AMERICAN DIET) TRUTH

Until very recently, the idea of food as medicine has been profoundly dismissed by our culture in a myriad of ways. Although the Academy of Sciences in the U.S. declared nutrition a science only 35 years ago, the Chinese have considered it a primary medicinal therapy for thousands of years.

In 1976, the United States Senate published a comprehensive study on nutrition, based on the testimony of 1100 scientists from eight countries. The Select Committee on Nutrition and Human Needs, chaired by then Senator George McGovern, concluded that much of the sickness and disease in the US. was directly linked to diet. The most indicting testimony came from Dr. D. Mark Hegstead, head of the Harvard School of Public Health. Hegstead claimed that six of the leading 10 causes of premature death in the US. are the direct result of the Standard American Diet, appropriately referred to as S.A.D. In the past two decades since the Senate Committee convened, a tremendous amount of research has confirmed and expanded its findings. Today, despite the fact that the majority of Americans have yet to embrace the idea that diet is fundamental to health, a growing segment of the population is getting the message.

Perhaps we need a reality check to realize how much our diets have changed since our parents or grandparents were kids. In the past century, the composition of the average diet in the U.S. has degenerated radically. The complex carbohydrates (fruit, vegetables, legumes, and grain products) which were the mainstay of our grandparents' diets now play a minor role. Remember, fast-food hamburger-and-French-fries places didn't come on the scene until the late 60's. Nor did we have the massive number of convenience foods, packed with processed fats, sugars, and salt, that we have today. As a result, the consumption of saturated fats and sugar has risen to the point where these two dietary elements alone comprise at least 60% of the total caloric intake of Americans.

This amounts to a wave of malnutrition, both over- and under-consumption. The over-consumption of saturated and animal fat in particular is generally accepted as responsible for six of the leading 10 causes of untimely death, among them heart disease, cancer, cerebrovascular disease, diabetes, and atherosclerosis. On the other hand, the under-consumption of good sources of low-fat protein, essential fatty acids, and complex carbohydrates, including fruits and vegetables, deprives the body of the essential nutrients it needs. This is particularly disturbing when you consider that today's children have had this type of diet from day one; they were born into the world of drive-through dining and processed, convenience foods.

According to a medical study earlier this decade in Baltimore County, Maryland, 35% of America's school children have high cholesterol levels. This alarming fact was supported by the well-known Bogaloosa Heart Study in Bogaloosa, Louisiana, which concluded that fifty percent of the nation will die of heart disease if the current diets of school children remain the same. And, Dr. Peter Kwiterovitch, founder of the Family Nutrition Education Program at Johns Hopkins Medical School, has stated that "proper diet could cut heart disease in America by fifty percent."

## NUTRITIONAL THERAPY

Today, more than ever, we know that food is capable of either causing disease or cultivating health. After such a long time in the closet, the medicinal qualities of food have finally begun to be recognized by Western science. More than 6,000 studies each year, funded largely by governments and prestigious universities, research the effects of various micro-nutrients in the foods we eat. Ancient Chinese medicine, and other alternative medicines that emphasize food as a primary healing therapy, are no longer considered "far-out." Researchers have isolated a wide range of medicinal and preventative properties associated with foods that can eliminate or alleviate a wide range of both chronic and acute diseases. On a cellular level, where all the action takes place, foods can act as cholesterol antagonists, anti-inflammatories, cell insulators, relaxants, antibiotics, laxatives, cancer fighters, and hormone stimulators, to name a few.

It seems that almost every day newspaper headlines report a new study establishing the role of a particular food in the prevention or reversal of a disease. There are some far-reaching implications in this research. Science is discovering the antioxidant, anti-cancer properties of cruciferous vegetables (broccoli, cabbage, Brussels sprouts and cauliflower), the heart-healthy (and other beneficial) properties of various unsaturated fatty acids including those found in raw, unprocessed olive oil and cold water fishes, and, most recently, the role of soy bean products as protection against a variety of diseases, including a host of cancers and heart disease.

Our bodies are maintained by thousands of processes more intricate than science can fully grasp: the intelligence encoded in a single strand of our DNA is too detailed for our best computers to unravel in a lifetime. Clearly, the human body is a wondrous organism whose many biological miracles are impossible without the right food.

## PROTEINS

Proteins, for instance, have a number of functions. After water, they are the body's most plentiful and fundamental substance. Proteins are the major building blocks that create muscles, tissues, blood, and the internal organs. Proteins insulate cells, protecting them from invasion by bacteria, germs, and viruses. They are also the basic ingredients of enzymes and antibodies—an integral part of the immune response. I think of proteins as the Department of Public Works; they do all the repair work of the body's basic infrastructure. When a cut finger needs to be healed, when the immune system needs to be replenished, when cells are damaged from a virus, it is protein that does the job. Without protein, we don't recover from fatigue, illness, jet-lag, allergies, or any biological wear and tear.

## CARBOHYDRATES

Carbohydrates, the second major nutritional building block, create glucose, or blood sugar, which acts as fuel for the cells. Carbohydrates provide our most basic energy; without them we have no fuel to support movement.

I break this group down into two fundamental types of carbohydrates: *processed* carbohydrates, such as table sugars and commercial bakery products, and *unprocessed* carbohydrates, which include fruits, vegetables, grains, legumes, and the natural sugars found in fruit. Then, I further divide both processed and unprocessed carbohydrates into high-starch and low-starch groups. Most processed carbohydrates are high-starch foods, while unprocessed carbohydrates include a large variety of both low-starch and high-starch foods. (Low-starch foods are those whose total caloric concentrations are comprised of 0-30% starch. High-starch foods are those with a total caloric concentration of 30%-100% starch).

The body reacts very differently to these two types of carbohydrates. High-starch carbohydrates enter into the blood the fastest, due to their high glucose (sugar) levels. This causes an increase in the production of insulin (a hormone) which, in turn, triggers a release of an enzyme called Delta 5

Desaturase which increases the absorption of arachadonic fatty acid. Arachadonic fatty acid, then, increases the circulation of another hormone called thromboxane A2, which increases the clotting factor of blood and causes vaso-constriction in the arteries.

Simply put, high-starch carbohydrates cause the body to store and maintain fat. They thus enhance the risk of weight gain and the accumulation of excess fatty tissue. They also increase the risk of developing heart disease, especially arterially-induced heart disease, such as atherosclerosis, which is a narrowing of the arterial wall. Additionally, after high levels of insulin are released in the blood stream, sugar levels drop dramatically. This extreme yo-yo action back and forth between high and low blood sugar can ultimately contribute to a variety of diseases, including hypoglycemia and diabetes.

Low-starch carbohydrates, on the other hand, have what I call a low *starch index*, which means they convert into sugar slowly and efficiently. They include such unprocessed carbohydrates as broccoli, green leafy vegetables, celery, cabbage, cauliflower, asparagus, and zucchini. High-starch, unprocessed carbohydrates include such foods as carrots, potatoes, peas, corn, bananas, and plums.

I strongly recommend that low-starch, unprocessed carbohydrates should form the largest part of your daily diet. Not only will they give you a balanced source of abundant energy, but they contain a host of healthy micro-nutrients and will not convert to fat as readily as high-starch carbohydrates.

*Low-starch, unprocessed carbohydrates*
*should form the largest part of your daily diet.*

This is not to say that low-starch, unprocessed carbohydrates are preferable for all people all the time. It is important
to remember the bio-individuality of each and every person.
While high-starch, unprocessed carbohydrates can be a problem for the overweight or diabetic, they can be nourishing for
other Constitutional Types.

Additionally, although a high-starch, unprocessed carbohydrate, such as a carrot, may have a starch (sugar) index as
high as table sugar, it has a much different effect on the body
than table sugar does. This difference has to do with the fact
that sugar is a highly processed, "dead" food, while a carrot is
a "living" food. "Living" foods are packed with enzymes
which are responsible for expediting a number of biological
processes ranging from digestion to immunity.  Although
sugar, a high-starch, processed carbohydrate, and carrots, a
high-starch, unprocessed carbohydrate, have a similar starch
composition, they are significantly different on the energetic
level. Just as identical twins have the same DNA but different
souls, processed or "dead" foods have a different energy from
that of a "living" food, such as a carrot. Additionally, living
foods typically contain other nutrients that help the body
digest them, as well as fiber which protects against many diseases, including cancers.

As a general rule, I recommend that people reduce or
eliminate their use of both processed and high-starch carbohydrates, and increase their intake of unprocessed and low-starch
carbohydrates, especially those that are "living." I will delve
more deeply into the energetic aspect of foods in the chapters
on the Five Constitutional Types and Food Flavors.

## A PATIENT STORY

No single food element is more addictive than starch,
and no nutritional restriction is more unpopular. However,

overeating high-starch foods can become a very serious problem if not properly managed. I would say that as much as 50% of all heart disease originates here, yet this problem is almost universally unacknowledged.

One patient in particular who comes to mind is a classic example. Andrew, as I will call him, is an attorney from Boston who came to see me several years ago after having been medically diagnosed with arterial occlusions of 90%, 80%, and 60% in his three major arteries. The medical people were encouraging him to have open heart surgery. Desperate and confused, he told me he'd exercised vigorously for 90 minutes a day, several days a week, for the past six years. He went on to explain that he'd been a strict vegan, restricting all animal foods from his diet, for those same six years. He'd also cut all fats (butters, oils, mayonnaise, dairy products) out of his diet. How, he mused, could his arteries be so blocked when he followed such a healthy diet and lifestyle?

After evaluating Andrew thoroughly, I found that his diet was laden with starches. He was eating mostly healthy starches such as brown rice, beans, and bagels, but high starch nonetheless. It was clear to me that his starch load was contributing to what was surely a high insulin, high fat-conversion problem. I went on to tell him how these starches don't start out as fat on the plate, but convert to fat in the body — with the same potential dangers as any cholesterol.

I took Andrew off of the high-starch foods and put him on a low-starch, low fat, protein diet. This, along with some dramatic supplemental support, helped reverse his condition. Adding the proper oils (borage and flax oils), and having him reduce his stress levels (stress produces adrenaline which also triggers insulin) also helped turn his situation around.

## FATS

Fats are the last essential building block of life and the least appreciated or understood. Essential fat is a term used to refer to the large range of vegetable fats and oils in diet. As a food, fat is stored by the body for future energy needs. It also insulates and protects all cells, helps in the assimilation of proteins, normalizes bodily fluids, and much more. Fats can be divided into two broad groups: saturated and unsaturated. Within each of these categories, there are many different types. This is due to the fact that fats are comprised of long chains of fatty acids, which can take a variety of forms. Fundamentally, saturated fats are among the principle contributors to heart disease and a variety of other degenerative illnesses. They are most commonly found in fatty meats, dairy products, and processed junk foods. LDL or "bad" cholesterol, which has long been recognized as a major factor in arteriosclerosis, high blood pressure, and multiple sclerosis is one type of saturated fat. LDL cholesterol is found only in animal products, such as butter, cream, and fatty meats.

Another type of highly saturated fat called trans-saturated fatty acid or transfat, is potentially even more damaging than LDL cholesterol. Transfats are created by artificially hydrogenating liquid oils to make them firmer — as is the case with margarine. They are most commonly found in deep fried foods, such as french fries and bakery products.

One 14-year study at Harvard School of Public Health, called the *Nurse's Health Study*, involving 80,000 nurses and reported in the *New England Journal of Medicine* in November of 1997, found that each 5% increase in calories (of total daily calories) from saturated fat (such as that found in animal and dairy products) produced a 17% increase in the risk of coronary heart disease. Basically, this was nothing particularly new in the annals of research on saturated fat and the risk of heart disease. What was very important, however, were the findings on transfat and monounsaturated fat. Each 2% increase in calories (of total dietary calories) from transfat produced a 34% increase in the risk of coronary heart disease. Additionally, each 5% increase in calories (of total dietary calories) from monounsaturated fat (such as that found in olive oil and salmon) *reduced* the risk of coronary heart disease by 20%! As this and other studies continue to establish, many unsaturated fats, or essential fatty acids (EFAs) as they are called, may actually reduce the risk of heart disease, multiple sclerosis, high blood pressure, etc. These EFAs are divided into two types: polyunsaturated and monounsaturated. Both types of EFAs are found in vegetable and sea foods.

Among the most healthy EFAs are a group called Omega 3s, whose food sources include cold water fish such as salmon and tuna. Omega 3s are believed to be responsible for many activities such as reducing blood vessel constriction, blocking the cancer-causing and artery-blocking activities of free radicals, emulsifying fatty deposits in the blood and low-ering blood pressure. Omega 3s can also be found abundantly in flax seeds and their oil.

Olive oil is another monounsaturated EFA that is especially good for the heart. Among its functions, it lowers blood levels of LDLs (low density lipoproteins), or the bad cholesterol, while maintaining healthy levels of HDLs (high density lipoproteins), or the good cholesterol. (LDL cholesterol blocks arteries, while HDL cholesterol breaks up the blockages, emulsifies them, and flushes them out of the body.) Because olive oil is also more stable than other unsaturated EFAs, I recommend its use as a general, all around oil. It is important to remember to eat as much of your oil raw as you can, so as to preserve its health-giving qualities. EFAs also enhance immunity through their ability to thin the blood, expediting circulation and the transportation of oxygen throughout the system. Many researchers, most notably two-time Nobel Prize winner, Johanna Budwig, believe that low oxygen levels in the blood — the result of a diet high in saturated fats — is the genesis of all disease.

It's very important to note that fats are volatile, vulnerable to high cooking temperatures, and harmful manufacturing techniques, which often render a potentially good oil dangerous. When buying olive oil, make sure that it is labeled as First Cold-Pressed, Extra Virgin. With canola oil, make sure that it is labeled as cold-pressed or expeller-pressed.

Many of fat's most significant properties come from its ability to convert into a group of hormone-like substances called eicosanoids that regulate virtually all cellular activities including anti-inflammation and immuno-competency response, and blood clotting. The most well-known, health-producing eicosanoids the body manufactures from EFAs are prostaglandins. Prostaglandins are responsible for the production of enzymes which are catalysts for all vital processes. Prostaglandins are thus largely responsible for regulating all gland and organ functions, including circulatory health and energy production. They regulate proper immune function, inflammatory responses, vascular stability, blood clotting and brain functions. When prostaglandins are out of balance, serious health problems will occur.

There are three categories of prostaglandins (PGEs). $PGE_1$ prostaglandins are derived from linoleic acids, or LAs, (found in most fatty nuts and seeds, high starch grains, legumes, fruits and vegetables, as well as many animal products) and gamma linolenic acids, or GLAs (found in evening primrose oil, borage oil, and black currant seed oil. $PGE_2$ prostaglandins are derived from arachadonic acids, or AAs, found in meats, dairy, eggs and peanuts. $PGE_3$ prostaglandins are derived from eicosapentaenoic acids, or EPAs, as well as decosahexaenoic acids (DHAs), both found in fish.

These substances have a profound effect on your health. For example, if a person eats excesses of high starch carbohydrates such as brown rice, potatoes, and beans (as do many vegans), this might contribute to a potential Delta6 desaturase enzyme deficiency and it is this enzyme which is responsible for converting linoleic acids into gamma linolenic acids. When this conversion does not occur, the risk of cancer, heart disease, and other serious illnesses is increased.

Even with its complex needs and interrelated systems, the human body has an amazing adaptability and can survive on a variety of diets. Denied the essential substances it needs over long periods of time, however, the body loses particular functions and develops weakness, chronic illness, or life-threatening disease. As a nation we accept this as an inevitable part of life, but it isn't inevitable. It is interesting that we hear the reports about trans-saturated fatty acids or sugar yet we think it's not a problem. How could it be so unhealthy, we wonder when our parents have been eating sweets, saturated fats, processed flour products, and minimal quantities of fresh produce for as long as we can remember. They survived, didn't they? But we overlook the connection between their diets and the fact that they are also a generation collectively plagued by a variety of chronic illnesses we've simply come to accept as a natural part of the aging process. Nowhere in the present-day Western world, except for rare individuals, do we have models of the aged who are agile, healthy and free of degenerative disease. The fact remains, however, that if not for our ancient ancestors, we would have no pictures in our consciousness of the possibility of human beings living into old age in vibrant health.

How ironic that we who have such relative wealth and

the choices that wealth bestows, have been hurt rather than helped by our circumstances. Perhaps we can change the way we think about food. Now, with the crisis in medical costs and insurance escalating along with a rise in chronic illnesses, Western medicine is beginning to acknowledge what its science has been exploring for the past few decades — *food heals*. Perhaps this acknowledgment will help us to learn more about the foods we eat and inspire us to take better care of ourselves.

While I very definitely believe that there are basic dietary guidelines that can be of use to all people (see Chapter 14), I also believe that an individual's needs are in a constant state of flux. Needs also change at different times in a person's life. I use the Chinese Five Constitutional Types system to personalize the basic dietary guidelines, thereby customizing food plans for individuals. To find out your particular type and the corresponding foods that are particularly good for you, refer to the questionnaire and chapters 5-12 on the individual types: Wood, Fire, Earth, Metal and Water.

## NATURAL MEDICINES

Natural medicines — both herbs and supplements — are the second main cultivators of life-force energy in this book and I include them in several sections. Supplements are concentrated foods, and as such their use is indicated when a person needs more of a specific nutrient than the diet can provide. Vitamins and minerals perform hundreds of functions in the body, without which we wouldn't be able to live. Please see the last sections of chapters 7-11 as well as Chapter 16 for the specific uses of the natural medicines I recommend most frequently.

There is no doubt that supplements can be used to enhance the health of a healthy person and also as medicines to treat illnesses. Researchers at our finest university medical centers continue to conduct vast and thorough studies on the effects of vitamins and minerals in reversing and alleviating degenerative diseases. Supplemental vitamins and minerals are being used to prevent or combat a wide range of conditions including prostate cancer, atherosclerosis, arthritis, liver dysfunction, the symptoms of menopause, anemia, and free radical damage, to name a few. Each vitamin and mineral is known to perform a variety of cellular functions. When used medicinally, they can aid the body to regenerate, nourish, and detoxify various systems, organs, and processes which results in health.

By all accounts, every ancient culture since the beginning of time used remedies from the vegetable and herbal kingdoms. Every animal's instinct (including our ancestors) is to seek out the balancing and restorative energies found in barks, grasses, roots, weeds, and seeds. From each botanical family we find a wide range of medicinal compounds. The family of iron plants, for instance, is rich in iron, while the family of lime plants has large stores of calcium, phosphorous, and potassium.

The formal use of herbal medicine is generally believed to date back some five thousand years or more, originating in China, India, and Egypt. The ancient Greeks, Romans, and Persians used herbal medicines, as did the Native Americans and South American Indians. The Amazon is still a rich source of medicinal plant compounds, containing some 300,000 species of plant life. This is quite awesome when you consider that the world contains a total of only 50,000 species outside Amazonia.

The modern science of nutrition has established that medicinal herbs contain at least twelve active substances which give them their healing properties. Among them are volatile oils, flavinoids, tannins/coumarins, glycosides, silicic acids, saponins, mucilage, proteins, vitamins, minerals, enzymes and trace elements. Among their combined actions, they work as anti-inflammatories, expectorants, anti-bacterial and viral agents, circulatory agents, capillary strengtheners, laxatives, cardiac stimulators, detoxifiers, connective tissue strengtheners, blood purifiers, and lubricants, to name a few.

Today, because so many people are tired of the side effects of synthetic drugs, there is a resurgence of interest in herbal medicine. While our ancestors had little choice about which medicines to use, today we do. We can pick and choose among a variety of natural medicines, while also having the option to use pharmaceuticals only when, and if, we must. Many people use over-the-counter drugs such as ibuprofen, aspirin and other NSAIDS (non-steroidal anti-inflammatory drugs) on a daily basis without knowing that they can be dangerous. Here in the U.S., 33 million people spend 7.5 billion dollars a year on NSAIDS and 7,600 people die from adverse affects arising from their use, including liver toxicity. By the same token, few people know that willow bark, available in tablet form, is an effective natural alternative to aspirin. It is also no surprise that several herbs have become very popular in both Europe and the U.S. in recent years. Among them are Ginkgo Biloba, which boasts 100,000 new users per day globally. St. John's Wort, too, is very popular for the treatment of mild to moderate depression. Black Cohosh, which Native American tribes called "squaw vine" because it was so good for the "squaws," is being widely used as an alternative to hormone replacement therapy for many menopausal women. The list goes on.

You can refer to chapters 7-11 to see which natural medicines are especially suited to your unique needs. These chapters are based on the concept of bio-individuality — the tenet that individuals fall into one of several different constitutional types which each have a particular range of tendencies, strengths, weaknesses, and needs. To find out more about a certain medicine, you can also simply refer to Chapter 16, which takes a predominantly Western approach to the chemical and mechanical properties of particular supplements.

## MIND-BODY BEHAVIORAL MEDICINE

Finally, I explore Mind-Body Medicine in Chapters 12 and 17. As I've stressed throughout this book, wholistic medicine refers to those medical models that acknowledge imbalances in *both* the mind and the body when searching for the roots of disease. Wholistic medicine, therefore, integrates a wide array of disciplines, including both those that address the physical body directly and those that address the mental and emotional realms directly. Those disciplines that directly cultivate life-force by unblocking energy from the unseen realms are what I refer to as Mind-Body Medicine. These therapies are also used to reduce stress and expand consciousness. Among the Mind-Body techniques available today are many types of meditation, including moving meditations such as Ta'i Ch'i and Yoga, visualization techniques, prayer, and breath work.

Chinese medicine, perhaps the first wholistic medical model in recorded history, is a guiding principle in my practice. Much of my Mind-Body Medicine is an adaptation of their work, and stresses the importance of integrating the complementary opposites within ourselves: our minds and our hearts; our right and left brains; our child self and our parent self; our intellect and our intuition. Chapter 17 includes this teaching, as well as the script for a visualization exercise aimed at this type of integration.

Chapter 12 contains simple instructions for a short but

powerful series of Ta'i Ch'i exercises aimed at bringing a meditative state to the mind and the body.

And now, Chapter Four. We begin with an introduction to the Five Energies system with which we can start to tune into the vast cycles of change within and around us.

# PART 2

## THE ANCIENT EAST

# CHAPTER 4

# The Five Energies

The ancient Chinese believed that all of Nature was connected in one vast web of life. When they looked at the world and everything in it — people, weather patterns, emotional expression, developing illnesses, or learning processes — they saw similar energies at work. They also knew that their fortunes were closely linked with Nature's changes, and they developed highly sensitive instincts that helped them recognize even slight changes in their surroundings and circumstances.

To a much lesser extent, we moderns, too, respond to Nature's movements. If it's cold we dress warmly; when it's hot we seek out the shade; if it's rainy we dart between shelters. We also plan our activities around energetic changes in Nature. We might cancel a hike if it's dangerously humid, take a brisk walk on a cool, sunny day or stroll the beach slowly on a foggy Fall morning. Our emotions are affected by Nature, too. Often, the first warm days of Spring excite us so much we can hardly contain our enthusiasm for life. Winter, on the other hand, may make us feel just the opposite — quiet and subdued, ready to hunker down and sit tight during the long nights ahead.

The ancient Chinese defined and organized the energetic changes they saw in the universe by categorizing them. They used the symbols Yin and Yang as the simplest way to describe the continual transformation of energy that was evident in the world. Everywhere they looked — from night to day, full moon to new moon, empty stomach to full, or sad to happy — they saw the universe expanding and contracting, fluctuating back and forth between complementary opposites that they named Yin and Yang. In addition to Yin and Yang, the Chinese also used a system based on Five Energies to categorize the stages of change that they saw in the world around them.

The Five Energies represent a more detailed description of the stages of transformation encompassed by the opposites that Yin and Yang symbolize. Any phenomenon that is described in terms of Yin or Yang can also be more precisely described using one of the Five Energies. The Five Energies can be used to refer to the different stages of any process or phenomenon, including the seasons of the year, the times of day, and the phases of a person's life. For instance, while Winter and Summer can be categorized as Yin and Yang, Five Energies thinking further breaks down Winter's Yin energy into two parts — Metal and Water — and Summer's Yang energy into two parts — Wood and Fire. In the center is Earth, which represents a balance point between the extremes of Yin and Yang.

While Yin and Yang represent the concept of the cycling of any two polar opposites in Nature, they also describe and

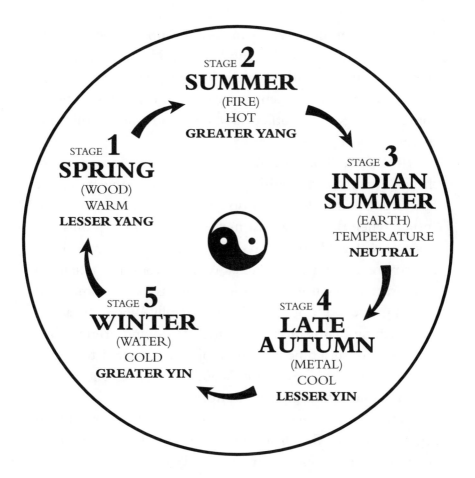

define two distinct energetic states of being. Yin, which we used to describe Winter's nature, can be used to describe anything or anyone whose energy is withdrawn, inward, contracted, consolidated, potential. Yang, on the other hand, is used to describe things that are extroverted, expanded, in full outward bloom — like the flowers of Summer. To really grasp what Yin and Yang mean, it is essential to understand that Yin and Yang exist only in relationship to each other; they are two sides of the same coin, just as night is the other side of day. One is not possible without the other, and they transform into each other over and over again, just as Summer gives way to Winter year after year. Put another way, ice, an extreme Yin energy, is bursting with Yang potential: it has nowhere to go but to turn to water. When the pendulum reaches its extreme point, it swings in the other direction. Contained within one energy lies its opposite.

The Five Energies, then, describe different phases of change. If we use the yearly cycle to illustrate this point, we can begin with Wood. Seasonally, Wood corresponds to Spring, when the ice has just melted and the first sprouts and green growth are bursting up toward the sun after having been in a contracted, dormant state all Winter. Wood takes many of its characteristics from the way Nature is at this time. It is planting time, both figuratively and literally. Wood characterizes anything that is fresh, new, enthusiastic, and original. It is a time of rebirth, a time to begin projects, to expand, to launch something new, to reach out. Wood symbolizes energy just stretching, unfurling, awakening from a long rest.

Fire Energy follows Wood and completes what was begun in Spring. Seasonally, Fire corresponds with Summer, when the sun is at its hottest and the days are long. The flowers and plants that were just beginning to sprout up and form buds in the Wood phase are now in full flower and bloom. Fire represents extreme Yang energy. It is the time to reach for our greatest potential, to stretch our limits, to expand our capacity. We can understand and recognize this energy in anything from the radiant and fiery personality of a person to the height of an argument, the passion of lovemaking, or the childbearing time in a woman's life.

Earth Energy comes next. Seasonally, Earth corresponds to late Summer-early Fall (or Indian Summer), the time of ripening and harvest. This energetic phase is characterized by a brief period of balance and rest where neither Yin nor Yang dominates. It is still warm but summertime is coming to an end. The days are beginning to shorten as the world starts to turn away from the sun. There is still some outward activity, yet at harvest time we begin to think about the Winter ahead. Although the fire of the afternoon's sun is hot, there is a chill in the morning air. This is the Earth phase, which represents an energetic state of being that is balanced between Yin and Yang. Earth characterizes anything that is in harmony, poised, and stable. Earth is the time to rest, to nurture, to unify, and enjoy.

Next, we have Metal. Seasonally, the Metal Energy corresponds to the Fall. At this time, all of life is beginning to withdraw and turn inward. We start to think about stocking up on supplies, storing root crops in the basement, chopping wood for Winter. If we're gardeners, we put the garden to bed for Winter, pulling up the dead plants and turning the earth before it is frozen and can no longer be worked. Squirrels scamper across the fallen leaves, gathering nuts for Winter. Metal is a time for reminiscing, reflecting, and analyzing what has gone before. It is a time for separating the wheat from the chaff, planning, and going inward. Metal can be used to describe a situation, person, time, or process that has these characteristics.

Finally, we have Water Energy. Seasonally, Water corresponds to Winter. In Winter, energy has reached its most internal, hidden state. While there is little outward activity in Winter, beneath the surface much is happening. It is a time of inner activity, internal fertility, and generation. Water restores and accumulates; it is extreme Yin. Winter is a quiet, calm time when feelings run deep and everything awaits release. It is a time for strengthening, storing, and rebuilding the energy that has been spent.

As we become aware of the Five Energies, we will begin

to see them at work in the world. Through this awareness we can start to recognize the subtle energies all around us. Seeing and defining these forces of Nature in ourselves helps us find our connection to the greater whole and our place in the world. We are, indeed, a part of something bigger than ourselves.

# CHAPTER 5

# Introduction to the Five Constitutional Types: Establishing Bio-individuality

Although you might like reishi mushrooms, I don't. In fact, they're not good for me, though they are undoubtedly good for some people. Similarly, while a mid-winter visit to Arizona would be healing for one person suffering through a cold and damp New England winter, it would aggravate the dry cough of another. All of us have unique constitutions with whole sets of different needs, tendencies, talents, and weaknesses; what is good for one can be bad for another. The Five Constitutional Types, an outgrowth of the Five Energies, is based on this idea. Similar to many other ancient healing systems, the Five Constitutional Types system classifies people according to their different constitutions. Knowing our Type — Wood, Fire, Earth, Metal or Water — allows us to key into who we are inside and how we fit into the world. Knowing who we are helps us focus on the kinds of foods, natural medicines and inner changes that are best for us.

The use of the Five Constitutional Types as a medical model for treating people according to their particular constitution is not unique to ancient Chinese medicine. Arabic medicine, classical Greek medicine, and the Ayurvedic system of ancient India all held that there were different constitutional types of people. Perhaps the most well-known of these systems was the Arabic which classified human beings into four types — Sanguine, Choleric, Melancholic and Phlegmatic — which roughly correspond to the Chinese Wood, Fire, Metal and Water Types. The ancient Greeks, too, believed that all illness was merely the loss of life-force that resulted from an imbalance in the fundamental elements: blood, phlegm, yellow and black biles. And the Ayurvedic system of ancient India distinguishes between three basic constitutions — Vata, Pitta and Kapha — which combine to produce ten possible individual types.

The most fundamental principle of the ancient philosophies that produced these systems was the idea that human beings were cosmologically intertwined with Nature. Living in harmony with the natural world was considered essential for health and prosperity. Ancient Chinese healers used the Five Energies to discover how their patients interacted with the world. To do this, they had to take the time to probe all areas of the person's life — the physical, mental, emotional, and spiritual factors that revealed his or her individual "energetic personality" or Type. Although individuals can be classified as a purely dominant single Type (such as Fire or Water), more frequently people are a combination of two of the five Types. For instance, a person could be thought of as a Metal-Water Type or an Earth-Wood Type. (You can determine which Type you are by filling out the questionnaire in Chapter 6.)

While each of us has a particular constitutional Type, we also have all the other Types within us in less dominant roles. For instance, a Fire Type (someone with a strong will and fiery, passionate nature) may have Earth characteristics when it comes to his or her mental capacities, or a love nature that is dominated by Water characteristics.

It is important to realize that each of the Five Constitutional Types represents functional processes fundamental to all human beings. While each of us has a dominant Type, we also have all the other Types within us in less dominant roles. Even though the desert is mostly dry, it also experiences all the other weather conditions known on Earth to various degrees. This is the way it is with us, too. As we become familiar with the natural energies that the Five Types represent, we will learn more about the natural world, including the natural world within us — or human nature.

Everything you do reveals who you are. *You* adapt to things that come your way differently than someone else. How you process particular foods, how you store fat, metabolize carbohydrates, how you respond to angry words or react to various types of weather conditions are all clues to your basic constitution. Knowing your Type can guide both you and your therapist or doctor toward the foods, herbs, activities, stress reduction techniques and climates that are best for you. Knowing your mind-body Type also helps you to stay away from the things that weaken your basic nature. Being aware of your predisposition to various types of conditions — your weaknesses and strengths — allows you to adapt to your environment in a positive, health-giving manner.

Knowing our mind-body Type helps us to see ourselves in an expanded way. Too often the effect of our society's one-size-fits-all thinking diminishes our sense of self. If we don't fit into the cultural ideal, we may judge ourselves to be lacking. By becoming aware of the concept of individual differences that the Five Constitutional Types represent, we can begin to celebrate the spirit of connectedness and diversity that the ancients understood so well. By learning about our individual gifts and talents, we can begin to see ourselves and others for who we really are, accepting our differences. Working with the Five Constitutional Types can help us to figure out who we are, why we're doing what we're doing and what we can do to make the most of the gifts we have been given.

## THE FIVE CONSTITUTIONAL TYPES AND CORRESPONDING INFLUENCES

The ancient Chinese were extremely knowledgeable about the natural forces in the world and the intricate ways in which they interacted with each other and human beings. This knowledge was consolidated and detailed in the Five Energies system. Each of the Types corresponds to, or rules, an array of things and experiences. These correspondences include "pernicious" (damaging) influences, food flavors, emotions, bodily organs, times of the day, and so on. In fact, everything in the world can be said to correspond to one or another of the Types.

## THE FIVE CONSTITUTIONAL TYPES AND THE PERNICIOUS INFLUENCES

Each Human Type is most vulnerable to one or more natural phenomena that have the potential to create illness. These phenomena are called "pernicious" influences and can result in a variety of symptoms, which we shall explore in the following chapters on the individual Constitutional Types. Basically, it is important to grasp the general effect of these energetic influences, so that we can learn to work with them. The ancient Chinese believed that the pernicious (or damaging) influences arose as a result of either emotional, lifestyle or environmental factors. They also classified pernicious influences as either *internally* or *externally* generated.

The predominant "pernicious" *internal* influences were emotional-mental imbalances. Consistently repressing emotions or obsessively dwelling on them was believed to result in internally generated illnesses, which would eventually create symptoms in the whole mind-body system — both internally and externally. (The emotions and their rulerships are explored later in this chapter.)

The *externally* generated "pernicious" influences were believed to be a result of environmental and climactic factors and include Wind, Dampness, Cold, Heat, Fire and Dryness. For example, Metal's dominant pernicious influence is Dryness. This can be seen in the way Metal Types frequently tend toward dry coughs, dry, flaky skin or maladies associated with a dryness of the internal organs. Because of this, Metal needs to find ways to counteract Dryness and create more dampness or moisture. Since this system of thinking is truly wholistic, it follows that anything dry would worsen a Dry condition. Therefore, Metal Types suffering with Dryness should avoid dry air (such as that produced by air conditioning or heating systems), dry climates, dry foods, and so on. Conversely, since excess Dryness hurts the already dry-tending Metal Type, Five Energies thinking holds that its opposite, moisture, will help balance it out and relieve the condition.

### ONE PATIENT'S STORY

A woman, whom I will call Laura, came to me complaining that every Autumn she got laryngitis no matter what she did. After a lengthy interview, we determined that she was a Metal Type. Metal, of course, is linked with the lungs which are responsible for hydrating the body. It's important to note that it was Autumn, when the weather is predominantly dry and aggravating for a Metal Type. On an energetic level, Laura couldn't tolerate the added dryness to her already excessively dry nature, and she got sick every year at this time. I suggested some simple changes that would counteract all the Dryness she was experiencing.

First, I suggested that she use a humidifier in her bedroom to moisten the air. I also recommended that she eat more soups and stews — vaporous foods — and that she spend more time in the bath or shower and take steam baths if she could or spend time in the pool room at the local YWCA or health club. I suggested, too, that she stay away from the pungent, spicy food group which has a drying effect on excessive Metal Types. Instead, I suggested that she eat more of the sour food group, which helps the body hold onto moisture.

I also discovered that Laura tended to have a lot of yeast infections in her lower body, in her intestines and vaginal areas. From this, I understood that she had excess moisture in her lower body while her upper body was excessively dry. This energetic polarization of conditions often happens; the lower body becomes too damp (with symptoms such as yeast infection or edema) because the upper body is too dry. In Laura's case, the excessive Dampness in her lower body was an ideal condition for yeast to grow, just as algae grows in a stagnant pond. I knew that we needed to get that moisture moving out and into her upper body. To do this, I suggested she stimulate the lower intestine by massaging it. I also encouraged her to release her repressed tears. All her life she had been the sad but stoic type, who rarely allowed herself to cry. But repressing grief causes an excess of 'overcharged' drying energy to be stored in the lungs.

Laura was very willing to make these changes and for the first time in many years she hasn't come down with laryngitis for two Autumns in a row.

## MORE ON THE PERNICIOUS (OR DAMAGING) INFLUENCES

In coming to recognize and counteract the pernicious influences, it is important to remember Chinese correspondent thinking — events and influences in the world (the macrocosm) correspond to events and influences in the little world or person (microcosm). Thus, the pernicious influences refer to the "climate" both inside and outside a person. The pernicious influence of Heat, for example, refers not only to high temperatures, but also to bad temper or hot flashes. Heat is also the condition of having too much activity, too much energy in an area, whether it be an organ, a section of the body or an emotional-mental experience. By the same token, the pernicious influence of Dampness not only refers to actual dampness (such as that found on a rainy or humid day) but also to excess mucus and phlegm in the body, as well as a lack of enthusiasm.

Remember, in Chinese medicine the reflection of good health in all the vital glands, organs, mind-body and spirit is referred to as harmony, whereas disease is referred to as disharmony. Harmony and wellness are the result of balancing the subtle energies inside and outside of us. A healthy balance in all things is the key to wellness. Here is a list of the Pernicious Influences and how they manifest in the environment as well as the mind-body.

### WIND:

Wind is active and therefore seen as a Yang phenomenon linked with the Wood Type and the Spring season. Wind manifests gently in Spring, hot in Summer, cold in Winter and dry in the Fall. The liver and spleen are most susceptible to the effects of Wind. Except for the Spring Wind which can be harmonious, Wind is seen as the most damaging of the pernicious influences. It is characterized not only by Wind outside in the world, but also by sudden change, often accompanied by a great sense of urgency. On the unseen (mental-emotional-spiritual) levels, Wind can manifest as sudden bad news, an abrupt encounter with rage or negativity, or a dramatic change in events. On the seen (physical) levels Wind manifests as sudden viral, bacterial or germ infections, sudden bowel changes, allergic reactions, and breathing difficulties. Additional examples of Wind include spasms, tremors, twitches, dizzy spells, convulsions, asthma attacks, fits of bronchitis, and sudden fever.

### FIRE:

Fire, both a major element and a pernicious influence, is an active or Yang phenomenon associated with all the elements. It is characterized by the feeling or appearance of great heat. The heart and small intestines are most susceptible to the detrimental effects of fire. Characteristic examples of Fire include hot flashes, heat stroke, boils, rashes, temper tantrums, relentless determination, strong will, and the personality of the 'Type A' workaholic. Fire often connotes an acute condition of some sort whereas Heat, which is similar to Fire, is often indicative of a chronic excess condition.

### HEAT:

Heat is an active, or Yang, influence often interchangeable with Fire. Heat can manifest as damp Heat in summer and dry Heat in the Autumn. The heart and small intestine are most susceptible to Heat. It is important to note that Heat can be the end result of an excess of any of the other pernicious influences. An example of this would be a pneumonia created by exposure to cold and wind turning into Heat, or a fever.

### DAMPNESS:

Dampness is a subtle energy and therefore considered a Yin phenomenon most commonly associated with the Earth Type and late Summer. Like all the pernicious influences, Dampness may manifest in any of the organ systems and may network its influence with other energies. The stomach and spleen, however, are most susceptible to its damaging effects. Dampness is characterized by a build-up of phlegm or mucous anywhere in the body, though it is most commonly seen in the spleen, stomach, lungs, lymph system and sinuses which cause colds, flu, viruses and allergic reactions. Dampness is also characterized by frequent urinary tract, kidney and yeast infections as well as excess acid in the large intestine. Depression, chronic or acute fatigue, lack of emotional expression and a diminished drive or desire are also characteristic of Dampness. Dampness tends to arise as a result of a stagnation of energy in the lower body, with a corresponding excess of energy in the upper body. For example, obsessive or compulsive thinking can pull excess mental or emotional energy to the head and upper body, leaving the lower body (intestines, bladder, kidneys, sex organs) damp and often cold from inactivity and stagnation.

### DRYNESS:

Dryness is a Yin phenomena linked with the Metal Type and the season of Autumn. It is most often characterized by excessive thirst, dehydrated skin and constipation. It may also be identified by pain in the lungs, or in the mid-thoracic and lower lumbar regions of the back. The lung and large intestine are most susceptible to the damaging effects of Dryness. If gone untreated for a period, Dryness will drain the Ch'i from the kidneys which are considered the body's reservoir. Therefore, those with excess Dryness can be understood to have deficient kidney energy. Since the kidneys are responsible for cooling the body, excessive Dryness indirectly hampers the body's ability to stay cool. Since excessive Heat is often a problem with the heart, it follows that Dryness affects the heart's energetic equilibrium. In this we see the way in which these pernicious influences move from one organ system to another. Therefore, excessive Dryness can cause kidney deficiency which can result in weaknesses of the lower spine, infertility, osteoporosis, frigidity, impotence, disc degeneration, cold extremities and a lack of stamina.

### COLD:

Cold is a Yin phenomenon most often associated with the Water Type and the Winter season. It is characterized by conditions that cause a profound chill or coldness to the body with a corresponding intolerance to Cold. Just as it does in Nature, Cold causes the body to contract, congeal and slow down. The kidney and bladder are most susceptible to Cold's effects, which blocks the digestive and immunological flow of Ch'i. Examples of Cold include chills, body aches, slow movement, lack of energy, poor circulation and even fever which can be the body's attempt to balance the excessive Cold influence. Cold can manifest as an emotional distancing or aloofness. Excessive Cold can result in the same set of symptoms as those associated with deficient kidney function, listed above.

## THE FIVE CONSTITUTIONAL TYPES AND CORRESPONDING ORGANS

The Five Energies thinking also posits that bodily organs and functions are ruled by the Five Energies. For instance, Metal is seen to rule the lung and large intestine, Fire the heart and small intestine, and so on. Metal is therefore seen to represent the bodily functions akin to the workings of the lung and large intestine. Since the lung is responsible for hydrating the body, Metal is then seen to govern the distribution of moisture in the body. Fire, with its rulership over the heart, represents the bodily functions akin to the workings of the heart, namely warming, spreading, and supporting. And so it goes.

Please refer to Chapters 7-11 for information on the five organ systems and the Constitutional Types with which they are linked. (Each Type is associated with both a Yin and a Yang organ. For the purposes of this book, however, we will be focusing our exploration on the Yin organ. For those who wish to delve more deeply into these teachings, please see the recommended readings in the back of the book.)

## THE FIVE CONSTITUTIONAL TYPES AND CORRESPONDING FOOD FLAVORS

As a nutritionist I have used the Five Constitutional Types extensively in relationship to the Five Food Flavors, or food groups. This aspect of Five Energies therapy teaches that each human Type benefits from a particular food group and is weakened by others. (See the Five Energies chart in chapter 2.) For example, the food flavor that is has a special affinity to Metal is pungent, which includes such foods as onions, leeks, garlic and scallions. These pungent foods are good for exhausted Metal Types since they are a vigorous food energy that, among other effects, improve circulation — including the circulation of moisture — which balances an exhausted Metal Type's tendency toward Dryness.

(Please refer to Chapters 7-11 for information on the Five Food Flavors and the Five Constitutional Types with which they are linked.)

## THE FIVE CONSTITUTIONAL TYPES AND THE FIVE EMOTIONS

Emotions, too, are linked with the Human Types. The ancient Chinese taught there were five basic emotions: joy, anger, sadness, fear and compassion. They believed that emotions were real energies that needed to be expressed externally and thus released. If, on the other hand, they were not fully realized and expressed, they would store in specific organs as unseen excess energy capable of imposing a negative influence on health.

For instance, unexpressed grief is thought to store in the lungs, fear in the kidneys, and so on. Since the body and mind work together, repressed emotion can often tip the balance overburdening a particular organ system, making it unable to cope with dietary excesses or other environmental stresses. Conversely, I've had many, many clients whose ailments have been relieved when they began to acknowledge their grief, or fear, or anger. Often, just telling them that emotions are legitimate energies that need to be expressed gives them permission to begin.

## THE FIVE CONSTITUTIONAL TYPES AND CORRESPONDING EMOTIONS

The **Wood Type** governs **anger**.
The **Fire Type** governs **joy**.
The **Earth Type** governs **anxiety**.
The **Metal Type** governs **grief**.
The **Water Type** governs **fear**.

Emotional pain needs to be understood in a more wholistic context in our society. Painful emotions are not a bad thing, nor do they mean that we've done something wrong or that we're weak. They are simply an inner reflection of a part of the true self that must be acknowledged and experienced if we want to be whole and healthy; in other words, after darkness comes the light, after grief comes joy. When emotions are acknowledged, their energy is freed to move and transform, rather than lodging in the organs of the body.

## THE FIVE CONSTITUTIONAL TYPES AS A WAY TO FIND BALANCE

In simplest terms, we're talking about a system that sees life as a mixture of vital elements and seeks to balance them to promote health and healing. Too much or too little of anything upsets balance and results in illness. So, on a fundamental level Five Energies healing, as embodied in the Five Constitutional Types, is a way to balance your individual blend of basic elements, including hot and cold, moist and dry, active and inactive, Yin and Yang. Five Energies thinking and the Five Constitutional Types not only open our minds to the idea balance in all things, but to the concept of adaptability. Like the flexible willow tree that bends in the wind while the mighty oak gets felled, we, too, will do well to develop such adaptability to change. Knowing and accepting who we are gives us a deeper understanding of how we can artfully adapt to life and live more harmoniously with the natural forces all around us.

To the ancient Chinese, adaptability was thought to be the most desirable of all human qualities. To be able to embrace ourselves and all things, rather than being contemptuous of what we're not or what has come our way, is a reflection of natural adaptability. To survive the inevitable losses and challenges that are an inevitable part of life on Earth, we must be able to adapt. If we can understand our energetic make-up — that we are particularly sensitive to cold, wind, or spicy food, or that fiery people make us feel anxious — then we can honor our sacred constitutional uniqueness and take care of ourselves accordingly.

# CHAPTER 6

# What Constitutional Type are You?

## *The Questionnaire*

There is no doubt that just as people are the same in many ways, we are also each different with varying needs. Although we are all subject to the same array of influences, each of us responds differently. *How* we express ourselves in response to emotions, *what* we're attracted to, *what* we dislike, and everything else we do makes us who we are. Although every human face is created out of the same elements, each of us is unique. This "infinite variety" that Shakespeare spoke of hints at the diversity of the natural world that is often masked by what seems, on the surface, to be the same. However, while each human being is a unique mix of characteristics, there are also strains of sameness that run through us. When you meet someone for the first time, you know, you *feel,* and you can often see how they are similar to someone else you know — or very different. Working with the Five Constitutional Types helps us distinguish who we are and how we are the same, or different, from others.

The following questionnaire is designed to determine your personal Constitutional Type. Frequently people discover that they are an equal mix of two of the Five Types, such as Earth–Water or Wood–Metal. In these cases, it is important to get to know each of the two Types that define your constitution. Our Constitutional Type is something that doesn't change, it is a fundamental part of our make-up that molds our choices and impulses, avenues of expression, tendencies, talents, and weaknesses.

While it is undeniably true that we have a dominant Constitutional Type, it is important to remember that no one is just one Constitutional Type. Each of us is influenced by all the Types to differing degrees. Remember, the Constitutional Types represent varying ways of being in the world, and while a Wood Type will be largely extroverted and active, he or she will also have a deep, introspective Water aspect somewhere within them. We are each made up of all of these energies, and it's important to recognize that their influence on us fluctuates. In one situation we may feel and act very much like our Constitutional Type, while another day, or in another situation, we may feel more like another Type. These energies are all within us and they wax and wane through time.

This system of Constitutional Types can be very useful used either very simply or probed more deeply to reveal a very intricate pattern inside you. On simplest level, it can be very helpful to realize, for instance, that you are a Fire Type who generates a great deal of excited energy which can easily exhaust you if not managed properly. It is most definitely useful for tailoring the basic dietary guidelines in Chapter 14 to your bio-individual needs. Should you become more deeply involved in this study, you can come to understand how the different parts of your mind-body flow together and affect each other in an intricate tapestry that offers deep insight into your personal uniqueness as well as the nature of life itself.

In any case, the primary goal is to determine our principle Constitutional Type. This is extremely vital to becoming our own self-empowered health-care manager. No matter what mix of conventional and complementary health care practitioners we may see in our lives, the ultimate responsibility for our health is our own. Knowing your primary Constitutional Type and acknowledging that people are all different are the first steps toward understanding the self. If you're going to be the doctor, you have to know the patient.

For each category, select the letter corresponding to the response which BEST describes you. For questions 1 and 4, please respond with an answer that best describes you during your formative and early adult years, even though you may no longer entirely fit that description.

1. **PHYSIQUE** *(in early adulthood)* <u>c</u>
    (a)   Square, well-defined frame
    (b)   Soft, round frame
    (c)   Broad, heavy frame
    (d)   Erect, medium build
    (e)   Thin, lean frame

2. **WEIGHT** <u>A</u>
    (a)   Average to five pounds overweight
    (b)   Five to 10 pounds overweight
    (c)   More than 10 pounds overweight
    (d)   More than 10 pounds underweight
    (e)   Average to 5 pounds underweight

### 3. COMPLEXION                                    *A*

    (a)   Slightly oily, thick and ruddy

    (b)   Very oily, burnt brown tint, and red cheeks

    (c)   Smooth sensitive, hydrated apricot tint

    (d)   Dry, thin, sallow

    (e)   Cold, clammy, pale white, thin skin

### 4. HAIR *(early adult years, your natural color)*      *C.*

    (a)   Dark brown, coarse, thick texture

    (b)   Red, reddish brown, coarse

    (c)   Medium brown, medium texture

    (d)   Blonde, platinum, white, light brown, thin texture

    (e)   Jet black, blue black, very thin

### 5. EYES                                          *B*

    (a)   Green, blue–green, hazel

    (b)   Dark brown

    (c)   Medium brown

    (d)   Pale blue, light brown

    (e)   Deep dark blue

### 6. APPETITE                                      *A*

    (a)   Very strong at mealtime

    (b)   Constant and strong

    (c)   Moderate at mealtime

    (d)   Light to moderate at mealtime

    (e)   Little to none

### 7. ELIMINATION                                   *B*

    (a)   Frequent constipation

    (b)   Normal with occasional constipation under stress

    (c)   Normal to slightly loose under duress

    (d)   Vascilate between diarrhea and constipation

    (e)   Frequent diarrhea

## 8. STAMINA

    (a)   Good energy, good endurance

    (b)   High energy, poor endurance

    (c)   Moderate energy, erratic endurance

    (d)   Low energy, poor endurance

    (e)   Very low energy, very poor endurance

## 9. PULSE *(Resting)*

    (a)   Quick and vibrant (70-80)

    (b)   Fast and irregular (80+)

    (c)   Moderate and even (60-70)

    (d)   Slow and deep (50-60)

    (e)   Very slow and shallow (40-50)

## 10. SLEEP HABITS

    (a)   Light sleeper

    (b)   Insomniac

    (c)   Sound sleeper

    (d)   Deep sleeper

    (e)   Sleep disturbed by frequent urination

## 11. MENTAL NATURE *(Positive, at your best)*

    (a)   Confident, independent

    (b)   Enthusiastic, exciting

    (c)   Supportive, caring

    (d)   Logical, precise

    (e)   Cautious, conservative

## 12. MENTAL NATURE *(Negative, at your worst)*

    (a)   Obstinate, argumentative

    (b)   Impulsive, consuming

    (c)   Meddlesome, manipulative

    (d)   Obsessive, ritualistic

    (e)   Stagnant, unexciting

### 13. EMOTIONAL NATURE (*Positive, at your best*)   *A*

(a) Kind, giving

(b) Joyous, optimistic

(c) Compassionate, warm

(d) Courageous, bold

(e) Calm, peaceful

### 14. EMOTIONAL NATURE (*Negative, at your worst*)   *A*

(a) Angry, impatient

(b) Vengeful, impulsive

(c) Anxious, dysfunctional

(d) Melancholic

(e) Fearful, disassociated

### 15. SPIRITUAL NATURE   *D*

(a) Agnostic

(b) Mystical

(c) Pantheistic

(d) Orthodox

(e) Unorthodox

### 16. SEXUAL NATURE   *A*

(a) Passionate

(b) Magnetic

(c) Passive

(d) Dispassionate

(e) Erotic

### 17. YOUR PERSONA IN FAMILY RELATIONSHIPS   *A*

(a) Performer

(b) Idealist

(c) Peacemaker

(d) Perfectionist

(e) Escapist

### 18. YOUR PERSONA IN ROMANTIC RELATIONSHIPS

*C*

(a) Loyal
(b) Tempestuous
(c) Warm
(d) Detached
(e) Mysterious

### 19. YOUR PERSONA UNDER STRESS

*A*

(a) Persistent
(b) Burned out
(c) Escapist
(d) Intellectualizing
(e) Avoiding

### 20. AFFINITY

*D/C*

(a) To be independent
(b) To feel pleasure
(c) To feel secure
(d) To have order
(e) To be left alone

### 21. AVERSION

*A*

(a) To be confined
(b) To feel bored
(c) To have to adapt to change
(d) To be spontaneous
(e) To be exposed

### 22. BASIC INSTINCT

*C/D*

(a) To assert yourself
(b) To attract others
(c) To be caring and nurturing
(d) To be organized
(e) To persevere

### 23. LIFE'S PURPOSE

(a)   To make an impact
(b)   To be loved
(c)   To make peace
(d)   To implement systems
(e)   To teach

### 24. POSITIVE ARCHETYPE

*(your ideal image of yourself)*

(a)   The Spartan
(b)   The Charismatic
(c)   The Mediator
(d)   The Organizer
(e)   The Genius

### 25. NEGATIVE ARCHETYPE

*(least desirable image)*

(a)   The Intimidator
(b)   The Egotist
(c)   The Manipulator
(d)   The Perfectionist
(e)   The Recluse

## MOST COMMON PHYSICAL SYMPTOMS

Circle only the most predominant symptoms/diagnoses in each lettered column below which you have experienced either acutely or chronically. Then total up the number of responses in each column, e.g., 6 under 'A' or 11 under 'C' and so forth.

## CATEGORY A

Abdomen feels hard after eating _____
Poor dietary discrimination _____
Feel gassy after eating _____
Crave fatty, heavy food _____
Acne _____
Dry, burning eyes _____
Muscle cramps _____
Tendonitis _____
Labile hypertension (acute situations) _____
Gall stones _____
Conjunctivitis _____
Hepatitis _____
Glaucoma _____
Meniere's Disease _____
Migraine headaches _____
Hormonal imbalances _____
Otitis _____
Impulsive, erratic behavior _____
Shingles _____
Mood swings _____
Photophobia _____
Blurred vision _____
Cysts _____
Endometriosis _____
Jaundice _____
Myasthenia Gravis _____
Lead poisoning _____
Toxic pesticide exposure _____
Gout _____
Alcoholism _____
Drug intoxication _____

**Total 'A' Responses** _____

## CATEGORY B

Acute upper digestive heartburn _____
Eating too fast _____
Feel hot and sweaty after eating _____
Crave foods often and constantly _____
Red, burning ears _____
Fever blisters on tongue _____
Varicose veins _____
Rheumatoid arthritis _____
Essential hypertension _____
Raynaud's Disease _____
Tachycardia _____
Hyperthyroidism _____
Heart arrythmia _____
Parkinson's Disease _____
Multiple Sclerosis _____
Hot flashes _____
Mastitis _____
Nervous condition _____
Fainting spells _____
Hypoglycemia _____
Low blood pressure _____
Acidosis _____
Adrenal insufficiency _____
Cerebral Palsy _____
Hyperactivity (ADD) _____
Phlebitis _____
Tremors _____
Day sweats (overheating) _____
Blood clots _____
Hypochondria _____
Angina _____

**Total 'B' Responses**                           0 _____

## CATEGORY C

Excessive phlegm following meals _____

Sugar and/or starch addictions ✓

Feel bloated after eating ✓

Crave sweets and starch _____

Tender, bloody gums _____

Fever blisters in mouth _____

Stiff, aching muscles ✓

Fibromyalgia ✓

Colitis _____

Gastric or duodenal ulcers _____

Gastritis _____

Chronic fatigue viruses _____

Enteritis _____

Anemia ✓

Hypothyroidism _____

Prolapses (stomach, intestines, uterus) _____

Hemorrhoids ✓

Diabetes _____

Nausea _____

Gum disease ✓

Bruise easily _____

Parasitosis _____

Athlete's foot _____

Candidiasis _____

Lyme's Disease _____

Pancreatic insufficiency _____

Mononucleosis _____

Anal fissures _____

Encephalopathy _____

Hodgekin's Disease _____

Epstein Barr virus _____

**Total 'C' Responses** 19

## CATEGORY D

Difficulty catching breath during meals          \_\_\_\_\_
Dietary discipline (a fussy eater)               \_\_\_\_\_
Nose, throat, sinus congestion after eating      \_\_\_\_\_
Crave hot and spicy food                         \_\_\_\_\_
Bed sores                                        \_\_\_\_\_
Loss of sense of smell                           \_\_\_\_\_
Pain with deep breath                            \_\_\_\_\_
Headaches with body aches                        \_\_\_\_\_
Asthma                                           \_\_\_\_\_
Bronchitis                                       \_\_\_\_\_
Emphysema                                        \_\_\_\_\_
Sinus infections                                 ✓
Allergies                                        ✓
Cystic Fibrosis                                  \_\_\_\_\_
Infrequent urination                            \_\_\_\_\_
Dehydration                                      \_\_\_\_\_
Nasal polyps                                     \_\_\_\_\_
Dry skin and hair                                \_\_\_\_\_
Sweaty palms and soles                          \_\_\_\_\_
Cold hands and feet                              \_\_\_\_\_
Sore throat                                      \_\_\_\_\_
Strep throat                                     \_\_\_\_\_
Tracheitis                                       \_\_\_\_\_
Tonsilitis                                       \_\_\_\_\_
Pharyngitis                                      \_\_\_\_\_
Mastoiditis                                      \_\_\_\_\_
Tuberculosis                                     \_\_\_\_\_
Adenoids                                         \_\_\_\_\_
Appendicitis                                     \_\_\_\_\_
Chrone's Disease                                 \_\_\_\_\_
Gingivitis                                       \_\_\_\_\_

**Total 'D' Responses**                          2

## CATEGORY E

| | |
|---|---|
| Little or no interest in food | _____ |
| Always the last to finish a meal | _____ |
| Feel faint after eating | _____ |
| Crave salty or crunchy foods | _____ |
| Dark circles under the eyes | _____ |
| Loss of sense of hearing | _____ |
| Lower back pain | _____ |
| Osteoporosis | _____ |
| Kidney stones | _____ |
| Cystitis | _____ |
| Edema (fluid retention) | _____ |
| Kidney/bladder infections | _____ |
| Lupus | _____ |
| Neprosis/Nephritis | _____ |
| Sexual infertility/impotence | _____ |
| Prostate disease | _____ |
| Urinary incontinence | _____ |
| Memory loss | _____ |
| Insomnia | _____ |
| Night sweats | _____ |
| Sensory or motor difficulties | _____ |
| Alkalosis | _____ |
| Enuresis | _____ |
| Syphilis | _____ |
| Anorexia | _____ |
| Gonorrhea | _____ |
| Scoliosis | _____ |
| Mercury poisoning | _____ |
| Bladder stones | _____ |
| Agoraphobia | _____ |
| Bulimia | _____ |

**Total 'E' Responses**    _____

Now total up all the occurrences of each letter from the characteristics and symptoms you've selected above. In other words,
see how many A's, how many B's, and so forth. The most
frequently occurring letter represents your Constitutional Type.
The letters correspond to the list of Types below. For example,
if the answer 'B' were the most frequently occurring letter,
then you would be a Fire Type. As I have mentioned earlier,
though, you will most likely be a combination of Types. The
goal of this questionnaire is to find out your dominant Type.

(a)  Wood
(b)  Fire
(c)  Earth
(d)  Metal
(e)  Water

CHAPTER 7

# Wood

Wood Types are as exciting and impetuous as the first erratic bursts of warm weather in Spring, as active as young children at play, as direct as the flight of an arrow. After the long confinement of Winter, when all outward activity is at a low, Spring bursts forth with an intense rash of expansive activity. Wood is linked with this season of rebirth and new beginnings, and, just as Spring fills the world with a riot of growth, so, too, are Wood Types eager to act, assert and thrust themselves head-on into life.

Wood is a yang energy, which means it is active and expansive, focused on expending itself into the world. This is the opposite side of the cycle from the yin energy of fall and winter when activity is concentrated beneath the surface and nature is quiet, restoring and replenishing itself.

The Wood Type, then, is assertive and straight-forward, as determined as the first green shoots bursting forth across dry

and barren fields. Wood is full of creativity, resourceful at finding a way to make things happen. They are enthusiastic and
forceful, filled with a sense that a new opportunity is just
around the corner. Wood Types are rough and rugged, strong,
engaged and engaging, busy and involved. There is never a
question about whether or not a Wood Type is around, you
will always know they are there.

Philosophizing and self-analysis is of little interest to this
type; it is not enough for Wood to believe in an idea intellec-
tually without doing something about it. Wood Types have a
tremendous drive to establish themselves through action and
are impatient unless they can move on their impulses. They are
fast and determined, capable of accomplishing a great deal.
No one is better able to initiate a project than the energetic
Wood Type.

Wood Types have a confident, positive attitude about
whatever they do. They love independence, putting great
value on liberty and freedom. Wood Types are honest, straight-
forward and impulsive, there is very little that is calculated or
hidden about them. They are naturally outgoing, with a strong
desire to stand out and be recognized for their achievements
and position in the community or environment within which
they operate. Wood Types strive to buck the odds, to be first at
whatever they do. Much of their strength comes from their
ability to persevere and work through whatever obstacles come
their way. They have great willpower and good endurance.

Wood Types tend to be adventurous, striking out to
blaze their own paths. They are expansive, always testing their
limits. They like the new, and tend to gravitate toward innovative projects that others overlook. They are highly motivated
and drive themselves hard.

Wood Types can be self-confident, bold and positive, and
they can also be stubborn and argumentative. When Wood

Types push themselves too far, they can spin out of control and become irritable and easily frustrated, lashing out in anger. They don't do well with sudden, unexpected circumstances or chaotic events, as their coping skills and adaptation are poor. Rather than finessing their way around obstacles they encounter, they tend to power their way through. Instead of stopping to pause and regroup, they charge ahead without thinking. While Wood Types can be great at getting a project off the ground, they can also become overbearing, not knowing when to quit. Too often Wood Types refuse to take the time to listen to others, letting their desire for immediate action get the better of them. If they are too impatient, they can scatter their energies and fail to complete the many tasks they have set for themselves.

As we've said, Wood Types are very active and forceful, tending to put out a lot of energy. Often their energy is focused so externally that they don't take the time to eat well or take care of themselves. When they are exhausted and need to keep moving, they can become vulnerable to abusing food, stimulants and alcohol without thinking. They live their lives with intensity, burning the candle at both ends; Wood Types are often the last to leave the party. Because of this, the Wood Type frequently crashes, burned out. This causes them to swing from extremely high to low; they are either going a hundred miles an hour or they stay in bed all week-end, depressed. To feel best, Wood Types need to find a way to temper their extremist tendencies.

## BASIC CHARACTERISTICS:
## A SNAPSHOT OF THE WOOD TYPE

Wood Types are generally average to above average in height with a square, athletic build and well-defined musculature. Frequently, they are five to 10 pounds overweight but rarely out of shape. Their complexions are often oily and thick-skinned, their hair dark brown and coarse. Their eyes are commonly blue or bluish-green with yellowish whites. They have a strong hearty appetite and good endurance. Their pulse tends to be quick, bounding and lively with an average 70-80 beats per minute. Their most common symptoms are vision and hearing impairment, headaches, high blood pressure and elevated cholesterol. Their habitual positive mental attitude is confident, while their negative mental attitude is obstinate and argumentative. Emotionally, they can swing from being kind and giving to being angry. They have a natural affinity for independence and an aversion to confinement. It is their basic instinct to circulate and their purpose to make an impact.

## WOOD AND THE BODY

*The **Wood Power** governs the liver and gall blader.*

Just as the Wood Type personality is great at "getting things going" in the outside world, the liver, with the adrenal cortex, is the organ responsible for "getting things going" in the mind-body. Through anaerobic glycolosis, or the processing and combustion of glucose, or sugar, the liver distributes energy through-out the body. In its role as the organ chiefly responsible for circulation, a healthy liver will supply the body with an even flow of blood, and can both store and pump blood to ensure an even release. The liver can be thought of literally as the Live-er — the one who mobilizes life and vitality in the body. The Chinese refer to the liver as the "General" who is responsible for sending the "troops" (energy) around the body for vitality, filtration, and revitalization. The liver is also understood as the regulator of the entire nervous system and it governs the functioning of the ligaments, muscles, tendons, and eyes.

When the Wood Type is firing smoothly and in balance,

everything is flowing and circulating well, just as a healthy liver sends a balanced flow of energy throughout the mind-body. When the liver is healthy, it tones, disperses, circulates and ventilates, keeping the system vital. It is the healthy inclination of both the liver and the Wood Type to circulate and move energy outward. If the liver is impaired, circulation will be cramped. In the mind–body this can cause little pockets of migrating inflammation and pain; fluid retention, or edema, especially in the face; blocked emotional or mental activity; as well as congested blood which can result in elevated cholesterol. Because of the liver's role in storing and releasing blood, impaired liver function is also closely associated with menstrual and gynecological problems.

The functioning of the liver can be "read" by observing the condition of the fingertips and nails; brittle nails and thin fingertips tell us something about the liver's functioning. Liver Ch'i also opens up to the eyes, so when the liver is healthy, the eyes read crystal clear. Conversely, if someone has yellowish or bloodshot eyes, it may reflect poor liver function.

## CHARACTERISTIC WOOD PROBLEMS

Not all livers are healthy all the time, and not all Wood Types are healthy all the time. When Wood Types aren't able to channel their energy outwardly in an assertive, committed manner, they tend to become erratic, ambivalent, contrary, arrogant and antagonistic, drawing their energy inward. In just this way, an unhealthy or out-of-balance liver impedes the flowing circulation of Ch'i throughout the body. This lack of circulation and congested Ch'i commonly causes an over accumulation of Heat, Dampness, and Wind in the Wood Type. These energetic imbalances in turn cause a variety of ailments, all of which are probable weaknesses and tendencies for the Wood Type.

While Wood Types exhibit good resistance to disorders of an acute nature, they are often riddled with chronic conditions. Commonly, these are a result of Wood's tendency to exhaust themselves by overindulging in excesses of all sorts, including emotional excesses, anger in particular. Since they tend to live life with such extravagance and intensity, they also tend to overdo everything, including their consumption of fats, sweets, spices and alcohol, which leaves them depleted.

Wood can suffer from restless sleep and carbohydrate metabolism deficiencies, such as low or high blood sugar. Alcohol addiction can also be a problem for Wood.

Depending on the particular time, Wood, like all the Types, can suffer either from an excess of high energy or an exhausted, low-energy state. These energetic swings are normal and affect everything in the natural world, including people. When Wood Types are experiencing a period of exhaustion or low-energy, they are typically vulnerable to a range of maladies such as these: cirrhosis; diabetes; chronic depression; blurred vision; low blood sugar; irritable bowel; neck and shoulder tension; cystitis; sound and light sensitivity. On the other hand, when this Type experiences periods of high energy, they are typically vulnerable to the following conditions: high blood pressure; boils; constipation; muscle cramps; ligament, tendon or muscle inflammation; tinnitus; cholesterol elevation; connective tissue diseases; eye and ear illnesses.

## A HEALING BALANCE FOR WOOD

### Sour: Wood's Primary Medicinal Food Flavor

The Sour Food Flavor is first drawn to the liver and gall bladder and is the most medicinal flavor for the Wood Type. Sour has a congealing effect that serves to bind or draw energy together. Perhaps the most specific conditions that benefit from Sour foods are cirrhosis of the liver and other similar degenerated tissue problems. Sour's binding, gathering qualities help heal damaged tissue by drawing it together, much like a lemon causes you to pucker your cheeks. In the same way, the sour foods have a gathering effect mentally, and can help those with unfocused mental concentration. When Wood Types are exhausted, their energy scattered and diffused, Sour can help to pull them back to center and reenergize them. Sour is also excellent for diminishing the craving for sweets. Any weakened, sallow, emaciated or melancholic, chronically fatigued conditions are especially helped by sour foods.

### Common examples of the Sour Food Group:

Apple, barley, blackberry, blueberry, Brussels sprouts, cabbage, cherry, grape, grapefruit, hawthorn berry, kiwi, nectarine, orange, pear, pineapple, raspberry, scallions, soy, strawberry, tangerine, tomato, yogurt.

## NATURAL MEDICINES FOR WOOD

### Barberry Root Tincture

Barberry root is a bitter herbal medicine. The more bitter an herb is, the more cleansing it is. Its bitterness is due to a healing phytochemical called *ilicin*. As the great naturopathic herbal practitioner, Dr. John Christopher once said, "The bitter, the better." Ilicin increases bile production in the liver/gall bladder region. This increases the alkalinity of the surrounding tissues since bile has a pH of between 7.6 and 8.6. With the increased stimulation of bile, the liver is better able to return to an alkaline state which allows this great detoxifying 'body filter' to do its job effectively—filtering out all of the accumulated toxins the body has ingested such as food additives, pesticides, and certain fats. Barberry is irreplaceable as a liver cleanser. I recommend dissolving 10-15 drops in 3 to 5 ounces of pure water and sipping the mixture three times daily on an empty stomach. Do this for every day for one month every six months. This is especially important for Wood Types who are careless with their diets.

### Chrysanthemum Flower Tea *(chrysanthemum morifolium)*

The Chinese call this popular herbal medicine Jua Hua and commonly recommend that it be used in the form of tea. Generally it is used to improve vision and relieve sore, tired eyes, but it is also often recommended for headaches associated with colds, flu, and allergies. Some studies in China suggest it is a useful herb for labile hypertension. Steep one tablespoon in a tea ball for 7-10 minutes to prepare a mug of tea 5 to 7 times a week.

### Coenzyme Q-10

For the past 20 years, bio-medical researchers have found hundreds of healing properties associated with this nutritional supplement. It has shown beneficial effects in treating a variety of conditions including obesity and especially heart disease. And while it has even been discussed as a sort of longevity enzyme in the American Journal of Cardiology★, I prefer to use it as a liver detoxifier. I have noted its distinct ability to release liver/gall bladder pressure, and as a result it helps relieve associated symptoms such as labile hypertension, sinus inflammation, migraine headaches, poor fat digestion,

---

★NOTE: When using homeopathic remedies, take nothing by mouth 10-15 minutes before or after dosage. Additionally, you should refrain from using coffee, alcohol, or mint products, including toothpastes containing mint, while taking homeopathic remedies. (Non-mint toothpastes are available at natural food stores.) If sensitive to alcohol, either use pill forms, or put drops in 3 oz. of warm water and allow one minute for the alcohol to evaporate. If using drops, place under tongue and hold for 10 seconds before swallowing. If using pills, do not handle them but rather dump them into the cap then toss into your mouth. Store homeopathics out of direct sunlight and keep them away from x-rays.

hormonal imbalance, irritability, and mood swings. I recommend a dosage of two 60 mg. capsules daily.

### Holly—Bach Flower Remedy tincture *(Aquifoliaceae)*

Not unlike Barberry, this is a superb liver tonic as it, too, is considered a bitter herb with high concentrations of ilicin. However, in its homeopathic form, Holly is a proven natural medicine for uncontrollable anger, rage, or temper tantrums. First formulated in the early 1930's by British physician, Edward Bach, Holly and the 36 other Bach Flower Remedies have been used successfully for decades by those seeking relief from a vast array of physical, emotional and spiritual difficulties. I recommend 3 drops be dissolved in 3 ounces water which you should sip 3 times a day on an empty stomach as needed.

### 5-HTP *(5 Hydroxytryptophan)*

This is a new natural supplement that has been described by many as Mother Nature's alternative to Prozac. 5-HTP dramatically improves the efficiency of the body's serotonin activity which regulates the body's sleep patterns and emotional state of mind. This supplement should not be confused with the Japanese tryptophan which was recalled in the late 1980's because of a manufacturing flaw. 5-HTP is a safe, over the counter supplement available at health food stores which can markedly improve the quality of sleep and the stability of moods, especially in the overstressed, overworked, excessive Wood Type. I recommend two 50 mg. capsules daily on an empty stomach.

### Linden Flower Tincture *(Tiliaceae)*

Over the centuries, Linden Flower has been used to treat a variety of illnesses. Among them are nervous disorders, sinus headaches, insomnia, and skin problems. In my work, I've found Linden Flower to be of great value in the treatment of various labile hypertensions. I've seen many Type-A personalities with substantial Wood constituents have great results with this natural medicine. It has the ability to take some of the excess charge out of an over-driven nervous mind and body. I recommend 15 drops in 3 ounces water three times a day on an empty stomach.

### Natrum Sulphuricum *(sulphate of sodium)*

This homeopathic medicine is a preeminent liver and gall bladder remedy. It has been used over the years for a variety of health problems including ear aches, sinusitis, conjunctivitis, and even spinal meningitis. This remedy is of great value for Wood Types with acute sinusitis, hepatitis, and chronic digestive gas. I recommend a 6c potency. Dissolve 3 pellets under the tongue three times per day on an empty stomach for one month.

### Choline *(Liquid Chloride)*

This supplement has been successfully used to support memory enhancement because of its proven ability to support brain synapse communication. However, in my work I most commonly use Choline (a B vitamin) to reduce blood fat levels (LDL or "bad" cholesterol and triglycerides). The high-living Wood Types who over-consume fatty, rich foods, alcohol, and sugars tend to do well with this natural supplement. Choline will also improve circulation, cardiovascular functioning, and memory. I recommend 1 tsp. three times a day with food. It also may be taken in juice.

### S.O.D. *(Super Oxide Dismutase)*

The fifth most common protein in the human body, S.O.D. is believed to be an anti-aging enzyme which controls the balance between oxygen and potentially dangerous free radicals. It aids the liver in its anti-inflammatory efforts, helps the liver with its detoxifying chores, and also protects liver cells from free radical damage and the dysfunctions caused by stress and poor diet. I recommend 1500 mcg. twice daily with food.

### Super Max EPA *(Eicosapentaenoic Acid)* in capsule form

Eicosapentaenoic Acid is what we call 'good' cholesterol. Current research has shown these fatty acids to be extremely effective in lowering "bad" cholesterol. However, the medical value extends far beyond cholesterol reduction. I have found EPA to be irreplaceable in reversing many chronic inflammatory diseases such as arthritis, fibromyalgia, and many forms of lupus. I recommend two capsules (225 mg. of EPA with 150 mg. DHA) three times a day with meals.

### ONE PATIENT'S STORY

I have been seeing Jay, who is predominantly a Wood Type, on and off for the past five years. He is a stockbroker in his late 30's. A well-known college athlete, he still plays tennis and is very active. He has a powerful, muscular build, and he is slightly overweight. His personality is big; he is very outgoing and can, on occasion, be domineering. He's a real Type-A personality — a high achiever, very dedicated to his work, intense, and fast-paced about everything.

When he first came to see me he was suffering from chronic constipation and muscle cramps that kept him up at night. He also had boils and other skin problems, especially in the spring and summer. Additionally, he had some ligament problems from old sports injuries. Because he was drawn to very rich foods — sugar, red meat, cheeses — his cholesterol and triglyceride levels were on the high side.

I put him on a low fat diet that centered on lightly steamed vegetables, lean proteins, and more vegetarian foods such as legumes and tofu. I suggested that he narrow his variety of foods, lower the volume and eat more fruits and vegetables during peak Fire season, which is summer. I also stressed that he should eat bitter vegetables, which are very good for reducing inflammation and calming the nervous system. To accompany the diet, I put him on a variety of Wood Type natural medicines, among them vitamins B6, B3, B5, CoQ 10, choline and inositol, calcium, magnesium, and potassium. He also took Linden Flower to help lower his blood pressure, and Holly (Bach Flower Remedy) for his mental tension. All of these were recommended in standard dosages.

Quite soon after making these dietary changes, Jay lost about 15-16 pounds with relative ease. His blood pressure decreased significantly as did his cholesterol levels, which went from the high 200's down to just over 200. His triglycerides, which had been consistently hovering at 130 to 140 mg. dl. when we first met, decreased to a around 80 mg. dl. His skin problems cleared up and he is now bothered much less by cramping and pain from the old ligament injuries. Jay has maintained this profile, and is in good shape now. He still has a tendency to overindulge in his old food choices and I think he would be better off if he could lose another five or six pounds, but these are choices that only he can make. All in all, he's in pretty good check.

## WOOD BREAKFAST #1

**Scrambled up Tofu with Soy Links**

> *1 lb. firm tofu*
> *1/2 tsp. oil*
> *1 small leek, diced*
> *2 scallions, sliced 1/4" thick*
> *Juice from 1 lime*
> *1/2 tsp. turmeric*

Mash tofu with a fork and add turmeric. Mix well. Warm oil on medium heat and sauté leeks and scallions until soft. Stir in tofu, lime juice and cook over low heat 3-5 minutes. Serve with lean tofu link sausages.

## WOOD BREAKFAST #2

**Warm and Fruity Salad**

> *1 chopped red or green apple*
> *3/4 cup organic strawberries, halved*
> *1/2 cup seedless red or green grapes*
> *1/2 cup blueberries*
> *1/2 cup raspberries or blackberries*
> *1/4 cup rice syrup or barley malt*
> *1-1/2 cup soy yogurt*

Combine apple, 1/2 cup strawberries, grapes, blueberries and either raspberries or blackberries. Puree 1/4 cup strawberries, rice syrup and soy yogurt to make a dressing. Stir as much dressing as desired into fruit and mix well. Warm slightly.

## WOOD BREAKFAST #3

### Creamy Barley with Soy Milk

*1 cup pearl barley*
*3-1/2 cup vanilla soy milk*
*1/4 tsp. ground cinnamon*

Add barley and cinnamon to soy milk in medium saucepan and bring to boil. Reduce heat, cover and cook until liquid is absorbed, approx. 25 min.

## WOOD LUNCH #1

### Pepper-Lime Chicken

*1 lb. free range chicken, cut into pieces*
*1/2 tsp. finely shredded organic lime peel*
*1/4 cup lime juice*
*1 tbsp. canola oil*
*1 tsp. freshly ground pepper*
*1 tsp. dried thyme*

Broil chicken for 20 min. Stir together lime peel, lime juice, oil, pepper, and thyme. Brush chicken with lime glaze. Broil for 5-15 min. more or until tender and no longer pink, brushing with glaze.

## WOOD LUNCH #2

### String Beans in a Spicy Yogurt Sauce

*1 lb. string beans*
*3 tbsp. plain soy yogurt*
*1 tsp. arrowroot*
*3 tbsp. water*
*3/4 tsp. ground mustard*
*3/4 tsp. ground cumin*
*1 tbsp. lemon or lime juice*

Steam beans for 10 min. Combine yogurt, ground mustard, arrowroot, cumin and either lemon or lime juice. Add 3 tbsp. water and mix well. Add yogurt mixture to beans and stir together. Cook covered and simmer 15 min. on low heat.

## WOOD LUNCH #3

### Tomato Lentil Soup

*1-3/4 cup uncooked lentils*
*1 cup cabbage*
*1 cup leeks*
*1 tsp. olive oil*
*8 cups water or broth*
*1 lb. can of tomatoes, chopped or crushed*
*2 tbsp. Bragg's Amino Liquid*

Rinse lentils well. Sauté cabbage and leeks in oil on medium heat until soft. Add broth or water, tomatoes and lentils to pot and bring to boil. Lower heat and simmer 45 minutes. Add Bragg and continue cooking 15 min.

## WOOD DINNER #1

### Orange Chicken

*1 tbsp. Bragg's Amino Liquid*
*4 tbsp. orange juice*
*2 tsp. arrowroot*
*2 whole med. chicken breasts*
*2 tbsp. oil*
*4 scallions, sliced into 1" pieces*
*1 tsp. barley malt (optional)*
*1/2 tsp. finely shredded orange peel*
*1 orange, peeled and sectioned*

Stir together Bragg's, orange juice, arrowroot and orange peel. Cut chicken into 1" pieces. Add oil to wok and cook on medium heat. Add scallions and stir fry for 3 min. Add chicken to wok, stir fry 2-3 min. Stir sauce and add to center of wok. Cook and stir until thick and bubbly. Stir in orange before serving.

*can also substitute pineapple for orange juice and add pineapple chunks at the end

## WOOD DINNER #2

### Beet and Carrot Salad

*1 cup escarole*
*1 cup romaine*
*1 cup beets*
*1 cup carrots*
*1 cup celery*
*6 rings red onion*
*1 tbsp. olive oil*
*2 tsp. Molkoson*
*1 tsp. Lemon juice*
*1 tsp. Honey*
*Dash ground pepper*

Combine all vegetables. Add dressing.

## WOOD DINNER #3

**Hawaiian Tofu and Vegetable Stir-Fry**

> *1 lb. drained tofu*
> *1 cup of cabbage, broccoli, bean sprouts, leeks, scallions,*
> *kohlrabi, Brussels sprouts, sliced thin*
> *1 tbsp. olive oil*
> *1/4 cup pineapple juice*
> *1 tbsp. Bragg's Amino Liquid*
> *2 garlic cloves, pressed*
> *1 tsp. fresh ginger root*
> *1 tsp. sesame oil*
> *1-2 tsp. arrowroot*

Slice tofu and vegetables into thin strips. Stir juice, Bragg's, garlic, ginger, sesame oil and arrowroot together. Heat olive oil over med./high heat and cook veggies. Add water if they start to stick. Add tofu and juice mixture and cook 2 additional minutes.

NOTE: *Consult with your physician before taking any natural food supplements.*

# CHAPTER 8

# Fire

Fire is as passionate as a young lover newly in love, as inspiring as a politician pounding his point home to a cheering crowd, as proud as a lioness with her young. Fire is linked with Summer when the sun reaches its most extreme point and in the Fire Type we see the fulfillment of Nature's most extreme potential. The buds and seedlings that were sprouting in Spring reach maturity in Fire's season, and the world is filled with fruit and flowers. Just as the sun is the center of our lives and we revolve around it, Fire Types naturally take center stage. Fire personalities are what we think of as hot-blooded; they are the people who get excited about everything and are exciting to be around. Just as the sun penetrates into every nook and cranny on Earth, Fire personalities radiate their consuming interest in life to all those they encounter.

Fire Types are very active; they are Yang in its most

extreme. The Fire Type has an intense nature with strong willpower. They are passionate, creative and emotionally energized. It isn't like a Fire Type to sit in the corner quietly reading by themselves; they are externally-focused. Fire Types are hyper-aware of their environment; thus, they are very affected by and susceptible to others, as well as intuitive about what others think and feel. They are generous and open-hearted, constantly involving themselves with others. They are comfortable with people and make friends easily. A Fire Type won't hesitate to offer advice to a perfect stranger, or suggest to someone what they should do in a given situation. If a Fire Type hears that you are going on a job interview, he will do everything in his power to help you prepare for it, and pump you up with confidence. They are almost always willing and able to respond to the needs of others.

Fire personalities live their lives with a strong emotional commitment and are very passionate about what they think and feel. Fire Types are easily moved by life and are open about their feelings. Where others see something as mundane, Fire sees all kinds of possibilities and exciting opportunities to explore. This quality, linked with Fire's extraordinary ability to communicate, makes them charismatic leaders able to inspire others with a transcendent vision of life. Fire Types are able to take the ordinary and make it seem extraordinary. Because of this, they often take a leadership role in their community. They make great politicians, teachers, CEO's of companies, entertainers, and the type of sales people who can sell ice in Winter.

Fire Types are enthusiastic, optimistic, confident, frank and outspoken. They have good senses of humor and are playful and affectionate. Fire Types are demonstrative and like to touch others. It's characteristic of a Fire Type to pat you on the back, put an arm around your shoulder, or pinch your cheeks. Fire Type faces are very expressive and their voices are loud as they hold forth in the center of a group.

While Fire Types are easy to have as friends, it can be hard for them to develop intimate relationships. They are idealistic and can be unrealistically romantic, distracted by images of ideal, unattainable love, while soulful, serious love can scare them off. It can be hard to be married to Fire Types, as their attention is so easily caught by what is going on just over your shoulder or across the room. It's possible for Fire Types to be unable to respond to the deep emotional needs of someone close, while at the same time they are caught up thinking about the greater good of society, or of any group with which they are involved.

While Fire Types have fertile imaginations able to dazzle the masses and sweep people away with their ideas and enthusiasm, but less fiery personalities may not entirely trust them. "Is she for real?" some may wonder. "Is he speaking the truth? Is he coming from the heart?" It's hard to know with Fire Types, since they may spark a discussion or situation just out of their need to avoid boredom.

Fire Types frequently tend to be Type-A, high-stress achievers who never seem to slow down physically, mentally or emotionally. They are often nervous and cannot relax. It is important for Fire Types to find an outlet so they can ventilate the excess energy they tend to accumulate. If they don't ventilate, or cool off, they easily build up too much internal Heat. If, for instance, they have a mild upset on Monday and don't do anything about it, you can bet there will be another upset on Tuesday. By Wednesday, if they haven't expressed their anger or frustration, they are likely to blow up. When Fire Types build up too much energy like this they can be overbearing and vengeful. Where a Wood Type gets angry and impatient, Fire can burn those around them with a blaze of rage that knows exactly where to strike to cause the greatest hurt.

## BASIC CHARACTERISTICS: A SNAPSHOT OF THE FIRE TYPE

Fire Types are average to above average in height with soft, round frames and limited muscle definition. They are often ten or more pounds overweight. They frequently have coarse brown hair with reddish highlights and coarse, reddish skin. When the ancients first established this system, they didn't know of any red-haired, freckled people or they would have seen Fire in them. The eyes of the Fire Type are generally dark brown with pinkish whites. Their appetites are strong and constant; their elimination generally good with a mild tendency toward constipation. Their energy is very high but their endurance is poor — they burn out easily. Their pulse is fast and irregular, generally 80-plus beats per minute. Their most common physical symptoms are cardiovascular problems, heart disease, angina, elevated cholesterol and atherosclerosis. Their positive mental nature is enthusiastic and exciting and their negative mental nature is impulsive and consuming. Their positive emotional nature is joyous and optimistic, while their negative emotional pole is vengeful and impulsive. Fire Types have an affinity for pleasure and an aversion to boredom. It is their basic instinct to consume and expand; their life purpose to attract love. Fire's positive archetype is the charismatic, their negative archetype the egoist.

## FIRE AND THE BODY

*The **Fire Power** rules the heart and small intestine.*

The heart is responsible for the movement of blood through the vessels of the body. It regulates the blood vessels, arteries, capillaries and blood flow "highway system" of the body. The heart works with the spleen to transform Ch'i from food into blood. The heart houses the "Shen," or spirit, and the internal "joy body." It is responsible for igniting the spark of life. If the heart isn't storing a balanced amount of spirit, it results in a whole range of mental-emotional-spiritual disorders. The spirit can be viewed through the eyes; when someone is manic, depressed or broken-hearted it can be seen in the eyes.

The ultimate visual diagnostic test for the heart is the complexion. If the skin has blue or purple tinges, this reveals stagnation in the arteries which reflects the condition of the heart. If the complexion is red, rosy or lustrous, it reflects a heart that is strong and healthy and good circulation of blood in the arteries and vessels. The Chinese say that the tongue is the mirror of the heart, and that a pale or purple tongue tells you that there is stagnant heart blood. If the tongue has an even red color, there is a good, balanced flow of blood through the arteries, veins and vessels.

## CHARACTERISTIC FIRE PROBLEMS

Fire needs to burn, and the Fire personalities must be plugged into projects and involvements so that they can channel their intense, excessive energy. Their most damaging imbalances result from a tendency to accumulate the pernicious influences of Heat and Dampness, and Fire Types typically suffer from excitability and feverish conditions. They have creative minds which are usually overactive, and regardless of how they appear on the outside, their emotions are never far from being out of control. Fire Types can easily accumulate excessive amounts of energy in their minds, hearts, and bodies. They are similar to Wood, but much more extreme. Typically, they are the Type-A personalities who need to slow down and find some quiet time to restore and regenerate their inner resources.

Fire burns hot and then burns out. Once exhausted of their reserves, Fire Types can become depressed and disappointed. Fire Types are so externally-focused that when they are depleted and unable to sustain their energy, and tend to lose themselves in the people, places and things around them.

Depending on changing conditions, Fire Types can swing from a high state of great excitement and expectation, to a low of disappointment and unfulfilled potential that leaves them feeling impotent and defeated. Where they were once confident and bold, they can become weak and withdrawn. It is important for Fire Types to seek out periods of solitude to help them temper their tendency toward extreme excitement. A sense of self-awareness can guide Fire Types to finding a balanced approach to life that helps them stay the middle ground more of the time and stabilize their tendency to swing to extremes. Depending on the particular time, Fire, like all the types, can suffer either from an excess of high-energy or an exhausted, low-energy state. These energetic swings are normal and affect everything in the natural world, including people.

When Fire Types are in an exhausted, low-energy period they are vulnerable to a range of maladies: adrenal insufficiency; slow, irregular heart pulse; low blood pressure; fainting; chronic fatigue; depression; premature ejaculation; pale, flushed cheeks; frequent chills; inability to concentrate; Reynaud's Syndrome and dizzy spells.

When, on the other hand, Fire Types are experiencing a high-energy period, they can become vulnerable to the following conditions: atherosclerosis; cardio-vascular disease; high cholesterol levels; excessive perspiration; irregular or rapid heartbeat; chest pain; burning, painful urination; cystitis; bladder infections; multiple sclerosis; Parkinson's Disease; rheumatoid arthritis; strong erratic pulse; pulmonary hypertension; eczema.

## A HEALING BALANCE FOR FIRE

### Bitter: Fire's Primary Medicinal Food Flavor

The bitter food group has special healing properties for all active (Yang) human types. It is particularly suited to the Fire Types. To the ancient Chinese, bitter is the flavor believed capable of releasing excess Heat from the body, reducing inflammation, settling down the nervous system, and drying water conditions, such as excess phlegm. It is therefore believed to have the ability to relieve hypertension, temper excess will power, disperse fluid retention, and freshen foul breath.

**Common Examples of the Bitter Food Group:**
Amaranth, arugula, asparagus, bean sprouts, beet greens, carrot tops, celery, chicory root, comfrey root, dandelion greens, escarole, globe artichoke, kale, mustard greens, okra, olive, papaya, peas, radish leaf, romaine lettuce, quinoa, rye, shellfish, turnip greens, watercress.

## NATURAL MEDICINES FOR FIRE

### Borage Oil *(capsule form)*

The prostaglandin action in Borage Oil has been shown to help regulate insulin levels which aids both hypoglycemia and diabetes. It has also demonstrated the ability to help many with multiple sclerosis, prostate inflammation, hormonal imbalances, and obesity. I have witnessed remarkable results when this substance is used therapeutically for hormonall problems in both men and women. I recommend 150–300 mg. daily.

### Calcium/Magnesium *(citrate)*

Both calcium and magnesium perform a myriad of vital functions in he human body. Among them are cell membrane permeability, energy production, blood clotting, and structural bone development. In Fire Types, however, nerve transmission and muscle relaxation are vital concerns. These two minerals calm highly stressed Fire Types, alkalize their acid-prone blood, aid in their relaxation, and improve sleep patterns. I recommend 1000 mg. calcium citrate and 500 mg. magnesium citrate daily.

### Flax Seeds

These contain a prostaglandin to go along with the Borage Oil. In this instance, it is better to take them in seed form rather than oil form to avoid the substance becoming rancid. However, the bulk oil is fine if freshness can be assumed. Nobel prize winning researcher, Johanna Budwig, lauds flax seed as having anti-cancer, anti-cholesterol, and anti-arthritic effects. My work has enabled me to appreciate its 'heart-smart' properties. It has consistently reversed dangerous cholesterol ratios while strengthening heart function. I am convinced this is a result of reversing damage caused by free radicals. I recommend that all Fire Types take either 3 tbsp. of seeds or 2 tbsp. of oil per day.

### Hawthorne Berry *(capsule form)*

This natural remedy has been used for a variety of ailments since the Middle Ages. The key active ingredients include bioflavanoids such as quercitin and rutin, as well as a host of proanthocyanidins. Its foremost use is as a 'cardiotonic' and a relaxant. Studies indicate that it also has a balancing effect on blood pressure — lowering it when it is too high, and vice versa. This supplement has been show to dilate blood vessels, thus increasing blood flow to the heart and its muscles. I use Hawthorne Berry as a cardio-tonic and blood pressure regulator and find it especially helpful for Fire Types who are out of balance. I recommend a dose of three 500mg. capsules per day taken on an empty stomach.

### Impatiens *(Impatiens Glandulifera)*

This homeopathic Bach Flower Remedy is a proven stabilizer for any irritability and impatience accompanying severe stress. This is a perfect natural medicine for highly stressed Fire Types. I recommend 3 tsp. in 3 ounces of water, sipped three times per day on an empty stomach.

### Kava Kava *(Piper methystrum)* in capsule form

This natural medicine from the South Pacific is a proven, 3000-year-old remedy for anxiety. A member of the pepper family, Kava Kava root contains medicinal plant compounds called Kavalactones which are powerful muscle relaxants and lessen tensions in the mind and body. I've found this most helpful for the highly anxious, panic-stricken Fire Type. I recommend 500-750 mg. per day on an empty stomach.

(Caution: this natural medicine may cause drowsiness and should never be used with any prescription medications. If you feel drowsy while using Kava Kava, do not operate a vehicle or any other machinery).

### L-Carnitine

This amino acid has consistently demonstrated the ability to dissolve bad cholesterol and other dangerous fatty arterial plaques. With the Fire Type's tendency toward heart disease, L–Carnitine is a natural medicine they respond to. It certainly gets my vote as *the* cholesterol terminator. I recommend 500mg. twice in the morning and twice again in the afternoon on an empty stomach.

### Potassium *(chelate capsules)*

Along with magnesium, potassium is one of the supreme heart-smart nutrients. Nutritional science has established that potassium helps the body regulate both the heartbeat and the blood pressure. Both the muscles and nerves of the heart are dependent on potassium for healthy functioning. Used with vitamin B6, potassium is also a superior diuretic. I recommend 99mg. of potassium chelate per day, and have found that Fire Types see superb results.

### NADH *(Nicotinamide Adenine Dinucleotide)*

Also known as coenzyme-1, NADH is an antioxidant derived from proteins and vitamin B3. Found in every cell in the human body, NADH increases the capacity of the cells to produce energy. It is one of the new supplement superstars which continues to show great promise in the area of healing the human nervous system. I am most excited about the research which suggests it may be of great potential healing value for many Parkinsons and Alzheimers patients. These and other depleted Fire Types may consider supplementing their diet with 10 mg. of NADH per day.

### TMG *(Trimethylglycine)*

Trimethylglycine TMG as it is often called, is a naturally occurring substance, a plant compound found most commonly in broccoli, brussels sprouts, beets, and swiss chard. A principal methyl donor, it has the ability to control Homocysteine, a substance many medical experts believe to be the number one cause of heart attack. Where previous research indicated folic acid as the foremost antagonist of Homocysteine, current research now tells us TMG is far superior. I recommend 300 mg. daily with meals.

## ONE PATIENT'S STORY

Donald, who is predominantly a Fire Type, is an Italian-American who owns his own business. He is on the short side, overweight, and not very athletic. He is very outgoing, charismatic, and aggressive. He gets excited easily and is exciting to be around. He's very enthusiastic about life and uses a lot of hand gestures when he speaks. I've had the opportunity to talk to a few of his employees who relate that he is good at inspiring and motivating people.

When he first came to me, he was troubled by excess perspiration which bothered and embarrassed him in public. He was also suffering from painful, burning urination, and very dry skin and eczema, which was worse in Fire's season, Summer. He was a classic case of excess Fire.

I devised a diet for him consisting of a lot of raw foods, especially in Summer, primarily salads and fruits. I suggested that he eat more vegetarian foods in general, with a target range of around 75% of his diet coming from those sources. I took him off red meat and fatty dairy products. I also suggested that he use a very low variety and volume of food.

To augment his diet, I put him on various vitamins and supplements: vitamin B1 for his nervous system and Type A personality; B6 for his urinary problems (he tends to retain water and B6 is a natural diuretic); and the B vitamin, inositol, a nerve tranquilizer that also has an emulsifying effect on fats. I also put him on choline to further emulsify fat and lower his high cholesterol and triglyceride levels, and potassium and magnesium to address some of his hypertension. I added the Bach Flower Remedy cherry plum, and aloe vera juice for hydrating the skin and the bowel to relieve constipation.

Donald was very disciplined about his new regime, and all his symptoms cleared up considerably He's lost 20 pounds and his physician took him off all of his pharmaceutical medication. I see him for a check-up once a year.

## FIRE BREAKFAST #1

**Minty Warm Amaranth**

> *1 carrot cut in half moons*
> *(slice horizontally down middle and slice thin)*
> *1/2 cup amaranth, rinsed and drained*
> *1 1/2 cup spring water*
> *1 spearmint herbal tea bag*

Combine amaranth, carrot and water in med. pan over high heat and bring to boil. Add tea bag to mixture. Cover, reduce heat and simmer 30-35 min. or until all liquid is absorbed and grain is creamy.

## FIRE BREAKFAST #2

**Pecan Rye Cereal**

> *1 cup whole rye berries*
> *2-1/2 cup water*
> *1/2 cup ground pecans*
> *1 tbsp. rice syrup*

Toast rye in 350°F oven for 10 min., and grind coarsely in blender. Bring water to boil and stir in rye. Add pecans. Reduce to low. Cover and simmer 30 minutes. Add rice syrup and serve warm.

### FIRE BREAKFAST #3

**Morning Quinoa Delight**

> *1 cup quinoa*
> *1 med. shredded carrot*
> *2 cups water or 2 cups vegetable or chicken broth*
> *2 celery stalks, 1 cup okra, sliced (optional)*
> *1 tsp. turmeric*
> *1 tbsp. water or olive oil*

Rinse quinoa thoroughly to remove saponin. Heat water or oil on med. heat and add okra, carrot and celery. Cook for 5 min. Add quinoa, water or broth and turmeric. Bring to boil. Cover and simmer for 15–20 min., or until water is absorbed.

### FIRE LUNCH #1

**Stir Fried Shrimp with Quinoa**

> *2 tbsp. water or olive oil*
> *1 bunch fresh asparagus, cut in 1" pieces*
> *2 large carrots, sliced into match sticks*
> *4 stalks celery, sliced*
> *1 lb. farm-raised, shelled, shrimp, deveined and rinsed*
> *1 tsp. coriander*
> *1 bunch watercress, rinsed and sliced into bite sized pieces*

Heat 1 tbsp. oil or water in wok. Stir fry carrots for 5 min., or until tender. Add asparagus and steam with additional tbsp. of water until tender. Add celery, shrimp and coriander. Stir fry for 3 minutes or until shrimp is cooked. Add watercress and serve over quinoa.

## FIRE LUNCH #2

### Red Lentil Stew

> *1 cup red lentils, rinsed*
> *4 cups broth or water*
> *3 carrots, chopped small*
> *1/2 dozen asparagus spears, chopped or*
> *beet greens, cut into small pieces*
> *1 lb. arugula or escarole*
> *2 tsp. ground cumin*
> *1 tbsp. fresh cilantro*
> *black pepper to taste*

Simmer water with red lentils and carrots for 30 min. Add asparagus, greens and cumin and simmer 10 min. Top with cilantro and pepper to taste.

## FIRE LUNCH #3

### Creamy Carrot Soup

> *1-1/2 carrots*
> *1/2 med. potato*
> *4 cup vegetable stock*
> *1/2 med. onion*
> *1 tsp. canola oil*
> *1/2-1 tbsp. finely chopped fresh ginger to taste*
> *Dash of dry sherry*
> *Dash of nutmeg*
> *Chopped fresh parsley or cilantro*

Peel and slice carrots and potato and put in pot with stock. Bring to boil, cover, reduce heat and boil gently until vegetables are tender, 30-45 min. Chop onion. Heat oil in skillet and add onion and ginger and sauté, stirring, just until onion is clear. Remove from heat. When carrots and potatoes are tender, add onion and ginger to pot mixture and cook 5 min. on medium heat. Puree in blender. Flavor with sherry and nutmeg. Serve with parsley or cilantro.

### FIRE DINNER #1

**Brussels Sprouts and Orange Salad**

> *1 tbs. olive oil*
> *2 tsp. Molkosan*
> *2 tsp. orange juice*
> *1 tsp. honey*
> *1 tsp. of ground ginger*
> *1 tsp. of grated orange rind*
> *a dash of pepper*
> *2 cups halved Brussels sprouts*
> *1 cup sliced fennel*
> *2 small oranges quartered*
> *2 cups watercress*
> *1 cup Mesclun Salad Mix*

Combine the first seven ingredients. Steam the Brussels sprouts for 10 minutes. Then rinse under cold water. Combine all the ingredients. Toss well. Serve.

### FIRE DINNER #2

**Broiled Cod with Mustard Greens**

> *4 oz. fresh cod*
> *Ginger juice from grated ginger root*
> *Canola oil*
> *Bragg's Amino Liquid*

Brush Bragg on fish. Rub juice from ginger and oil onto fish. Broil 10 min. per 1" thickness of fish or until it flakes with fork.

### Yellow Mustard Greens

*1 bunch mustard greens, chopped into small pieces*
*1 tbsp. olive oil*
*1 med. onion, sliced*
*1 leek, sliced*
*Turmeric*
*Bragg's Amino Liquid*

Heat oil over med. heat. Add onion, leek and sauté 2 min. Add greens and turmeric and sauté 8 min. Add water if needed and add Bragg to taste.

## FIRE DINNER #3

### Broccoli, Watercress and Mandarin Orange Salad

*1cup of sliced Mandarin oranges*
*2 cups of broccoli florets*
*1 cup of watercress*
*10 red onion rings*
*1 tbs. olive oil*
*2 tsp. of orange juice*
*1 tsp. of honey*
*2 tsp. of Molkosan*
*A dash of ground pepper*
*2 cups of tossed greens*
*1/2 cup Sliced Almonds*

Steam the broccoli 5-10 minutes. Rinse under cold water. Combine olive oil, honey, orange juice and Molkosan. Add broccoli, onion, orange sections and watercress to the sauce. Stir well. Spread over mixed greens and serve topped with sliced almonds.

NOTE: *Consult with your physician before taking any natural food supplements.*

# CHAPTER 9

# Earth

Earth is as sure and solid as the ground beneath your feet, as nurturing as a loving mother, as sustaining as a vast field of corn, as sheltering as the walls of a house. After the heat and fervent activity of the height of Summer comes a time of effortless ripening. Late summer-early Fall — the time of year linked with the Earth Type — is that in-between time of fulfillment and satisfaction. Earth represents this brief period of poise after the activity of Summer, but before Fall's harvest. This is the still point when the forces of day and night — Yin and Yang — are in perfect balance.

Earth is the only one of the Five Types that is neither predominantly Yin nor Yang, but a blending of the two. Therefore, it is both active and withdrawn, both outward and inward, both expansive and contracting. Earth Types, then, share this balanced energy. They are the peacemakers who like life best when everything is flowing smoothly. They are down to earth, cheerful, and pleasant to be around. They have an aversion to conflict and will do almost anything they can to keep events on an even keel. Earth Types are driven to bring everything into the center, to unify opposing factions and create a nice, safe, secure environment.

Earth Types are highly social and can be very relaxed and relaxing to be around. Through their love of people, Earth Types are able to instinctively identify with a wide range of individuals, drawing them in through a sense of shared values. In a group, they pull people together by focusing on what others have in common, rather than what divides them. This attitude serves to create and sustain relationships that might have floundered without the Earth Type's intervention. Earth Types feel most secure in a large group of people who are working together cooperatively. It is very important for this type to have a solid network of friends and family around them and they are often the glue that holds a group together. They derive much security from this sense of connection to the world. Earth Types crave security and feel for those who are without. They are therefore extremely compassionate and empathetic, always ready to lend a helping hand to those in need.

Earth Types are grounded and practical, concerned that life's everyday needs be met for those they love as well as themselves. Home is the center of an Earth Type's world, and they love to share it; food and homemaking are a big part of their lives. This Type also does well working at home. If they do work at an office, their work space will be filled with drawings and warm, homey details. They need to have a warm, comfortable atmosphere around them as much as possible.

Earth Types find their sense of place in the world through their placement in other people's lives and need to be useful to others. They have highly developed protective natures and seek to extend their blanket of protection across their friends and family. Earth Types do this by making things comfortable for others. They are the ones who send a container of food along to a new acquaintance, or offer to take care of the kids if you're busy, or make sure that your driveway has been plowed after a big storm. Earth Types take care of earthly things, and try always to make the world around them a comfortable place where things run smoothly. Unlike a Fire Type who takes center stage, Earth Types control the action from behind the scenes.

Like all the Constitutional Types, Earth Types manifest their energies differently depending on whether they're at their best or not. When their powerful need to keep their lives peaceful and harmonious gets out of hand, they tend to become very anxious. Sometimes, this can cause Earth Types to become manipulative and interfering as they attempt to control events and people. They are very concerned with security, safety, and groundedness; this can lead to excessive worry when situations are in flux and events seem uncertain. Often, Earth Types will search outside themselves for something to help them calm their worries. This dynamic often accounts for the Earth Type's addictive nature, which can involve the over-use and abuse of any number of behaviors and substances, from food to drugs.

## BASIC CHARACTERISTICS:
## A SNAPSHOT OF THE EARTH TYPE

Earth Types tend to have a roundish, thick frame and average height and weight. They have little muscle definition though their flesh is firm. They have a soft, hydrated complexion which can tend to be the puffy. Their hair is often medium brown and medium textured. Their appetite is usually moderate and their elimination is normal to slightly loose. Earth Types tend to have erratic energy, with moderate stamina, and endurance. They have an even pulse, generally between 60-70 beats per minute. Their most common illnesses often include swollen glands, chronic immune and digestive deficiencies. Their positive mental nature is supportive and caring; their negative mental nature is meddlesome and manipulative. Emotionally, they can swing from being compassionate and warm to being anxious and perhaps even agoraphobic. Their affinity is for security while they are averse to adaptation; they don't like change. It is their basic instinct to seek balance and their purpose to create peace. Their positive archetype is the mediator and their negative archetype is the manipulator.

### EARTH AND THE BODY

*The Earth Power governs the spleen and stomach.*

The spleen is the primary organ responsible for digestion, which involves extracting nutrients from food, distilling them, and transforming them into blood. How well it does its job results in either good or poor blood quality. When the spleen's function is impaired, there is fatigue, abdominal distention, and edema (fluid retention). Spleen impairment also results in a loss of immunological function, chronic viruses, swollen glands, tumors, burning stomach, candida, and loose bowels. The spleen is the organ that is affected by worry and anxiety, so too much of these emotions will burden it. A well-functioning spleen balances the mind. Food, through the functioning of the spleen, brings us "down to earth," balances us chemically, and has an overall harmonizing effect. The ancient Chinese believed that peace of mind was something that took place in both the mind and the body and was reflected in the blood. To their way of thinking, the spleen was responsible for transforming mental energy into a particular quality, or spirit, of blood.

## CHARACTERISTIC EARTH PROBLEMS

Earth Types have a moderately good appetite unless they are run down or ill. They have a distinct affinity for sweets and carbohydrates, which can become a problem for them. When they are stressed, they are prone to overeat sweets and starches as a way to fill themselves up. While a small amount of sweet food has a harmonizing effect on the Earth Type, too much can be damaging. It is also essential to understand that the ancients had no processed sugars or sugar products, so that sweet had a different meaning. Proteins, such as poultry, meats, and fish were considered sweet due to their metaphorically sweet nature as commodities that were rare and precious. (Please see the list of Sweet foods later in this chapter.) So too, a bit of sweet behavior — gift-giving for instance, goes far to soothe a troubled Earth Type.

Earth needs to guard against the tendency to accumulate Cold and Dampness; these pernicious influences are the most potentially damaging for them. Mucous and phlegm, manifestations of Dampness, can riddle the digestive system and the lymph glands. Edema, or fluid retention, also a manifestation of Dampness, is also a characteristic problem for the Earth Type.

Earth Types have only moderately good resistance to chronic ailments, which tend to manifest as spleen, lymphatic, and general immune dysfunction. These problems can result in chronic fatigue, frequent colds and flus, swollen glands, loose stools and erratic appetite. Earth Types sleep soundly, requiring at least eight hours a night or they run down their immune systems. When not troubled by anxiety, they are usually early risers. At their most vulnerable, Earth Types can become easily depressed and disinterested in life. They may also be intolerant of many foods, and highly sensitive to environmental conditions. Both their immune systems and their capacity to adapt to changing circumstances tend to be deficient.

Depending on the particular time, Earth, like all the Types, can suffer either from an excess of high energy or an exhausted, low-energy state. These energetic swings are normal and affect everything in the natural world, including people. When experiencing an exhausted, or low-energy period, Earth Types are vulnerable to the following conditions: swollen tissue; anemia; chronic fatigue syndrome; multiple chemical sensitivity; chronic allergies; lumps; tumors; acne; cysts; weak wrists and ankles; uterine and stomach polyps; varicose veins; slow wound healing; bloody gums; tooth decay; hyperthyroid; bloat; yeast infections; loose stools. When, on the other hand, this Type is experiencing a period of high-energy, they can become vulnerable to a range of maladies including conjunctivitis, uncontrollable appetite, panic and anxiety, water retention, PMS, mood swings, sugar cravings, upper body sores, puffy eyelids, leukemia, lymphatic cancer, stomach cancer, phlegmatic eyes, ears, nose and throat.

## A HEALING BALANCE FOR EARTH

### Sweet: Earth's Primary Medicinal Food Flavor

Limited, unconcentrated amounts of the Sweet foods will energize all Earth Types. This is especially true of Earth Types when they are in low energy, deficient periods. The ancient Chinese held that the Sweet flavor (not including processed sugars) aids the digestive processes, giving short-term strength to the stomach and spleen. Sweet can then both aid digestion and soothe the spirits, temporarily reversing feelings of anxiety, tension, and fatigue.

**Common Examples of the Sweet Food Group:**

Almond, apricot, avocado, bass, banana, beef, beets, beans, broccoli, cauliflower, cashew, chicken, cod, corn, dairy, date, fig, flounder, haddock, halibut, ham, honey, lamb, maple syrup, melon, millet, oat, peach, pork, potato, quinoa, raisins, rice, rice syrup, salmon, sesame seed, spinach, summer squash, sunflower seed, sweet potato, swordfish, trout, tuna, turkey, walnut, wheat, winter squash, zucchini.

NOTE: Certain protein foods, which are classified as Sweet Flavored, are better for some human types than others. For example: fattier proteins such as red meats, pork, ham, lamb, dark poultry, eggs and whole fat dairy products (whole milk, cheeses, sour cream, etc.) are best avoided by all active (Yang) Earth types, as well as all Wood and Fire Types. Most of the above mentioned flesh proteins may be better utilized from time to time by most deficient (Yin) Earth Types, as well as all Metal and Water Types. If using red meat, get very lean cuts, such as "dieter's lean" or top of the round cuts. If using eggs, it is best to poach or soft boil them. Lean proteins such as tofu, fish, and lean poultry are best for active (Yang) Earth Types, and all Wood and Fire Types. (I consider fatty dairy foods disadvantageous in general, and recommend that they be used sparingly).

## NATURAL MEDICINES FOR EARTH EXCESS

### Astragalus Membranaceus *(Leguminosae)*

Also called Ma Huang by the Chinese, this is the oldest and most widely used herbal tonic in Chinese medicine. They use it to strengthen the pericardium, or 'heart shield,' said to protect one from all incoming negative energies — ranging from "bad vibes" to viruses. Astragalus has consistently proven

itself on both sides of the ocean as an immune tonic. It fortifies immunity with spleen and lymph support, and has
demonstrated the ability to lessen both frequency and duration
of colds, flus, and allergy symptoms. I recommend 1200 mg.
per day on an empty stomach.

### Beta Carotene

This celebrated member of the carotenoid family has
clearly establish itself among the top substances for bolstering
the immune system. Scientists have been enamored with Beta
Carotene's pro-vitamin A activity, and have acknowledged that
it possesses an anti–tumor component. Extracted from food
sources such as carrots, acorn squash, and pumpkin, this
orange pigment concentrate has shown a great ability to
strengthen the immune system against everything from the
common cold to cancer. While recent research seems to suggest that some of its carotenoid family members (alpha
carotene and lycopene) are even more powerful, I am still an
avid supporter of this substance. I recommend 10,000 IU
(international units) per day as a food supplement to all of
those fresh orange and red vegetables!

### Chromium *GTF (Glucose Tolerance Factor)*

Most Earth Types have an affinity for sugars and sweet
desserts. The mineral chromium has the reputation as a sugar
appetite suppressant as it helps the pancreas to more efficiently regulate the release of insulin. This sugar-regulating mineral
is an especially potent energy modulator for most Earth Types.
I recommend 200 mcg. be taken with food at lunch time
once daily.

### Wild Siberian Ginseng *(Analiaceae)*

Ginseng is perhaps the most storied of all Chinese herbs.
Its therapeutic benefits have been lauded for nearly 8,000

years. As a tonic, it is especially noted for its ability to increase stamina and resistance to stress and disease. Wild Siberian Ginseng (also known as Ciwugia) is considered one of the most effective of all ginseng tonics. In recent years, it has gained attention for its powerful energizing effect on members of the U.S. Olympic team. I recommend 100 mg. of this supplement in capsule form twice a day on an empty stomach.

### Pau D'Arco *(Taheebo Lapacho)*

This South American tree bark has anti-bacterial, anti-fungal, and anti-viral properties. Most typically it is recommended for its anti-yeast capabilities. Earth Types have a strong tendency toward chronic candida yeast as a result of their over-consumption of sugar and starch. Thus, for most Earth Types I recommend one cup of Pau D'Arco tea once a day.

### Propolis

A bee resin collected from the poplar tree, this natural supplement gets my vote as the consummate immune tonic. According to history, Propolis was once used by the ancient army of Sparta to increase their strength and stamina before entering into combat. Recent research has shown Propolis' efficacy on an array of stubborn viruses and bacteria. I recommend a Propolis form known as Nordisk exclusively because I've seen what it can do first hand, especially for colds, flu, and allergy-prone Earth Types. I suggest one Nordisk Propolis capsule per day on an empty stomach.

### Red Clover *(Trifolium pratense)* *(Leguminosae)*

Red Clover has been used for everything from skin conditions to spasmodic coughs. I have come to appreciate its ability to keep the spleen and lymph system clean. Earth Types are general phlegmatic and would generally benefit from this pleasant tasting herb in tea form. I recommend one cup per day, and up to three cups for phlegm-producing colds, flu, and allergies.

### Vitamin E *(D-Alpha Tocopherol)*

Vitamin E is a well-known anti-oxidant which aids in the synthesis of DNA, RNA, and red blood cells. It also insulates cell membranes, protecting them from viruses, germs, bacteria, and free radical damage. I find it irreplaceable for most deficient Earth Types as an immuno-modulator. I recommend 400 IU per day with food.

### Vitamin B12 *(Cyanocobalamin)*

This vitamin helps the body synthesize DNA and red blood cells. Most importantly, for exhausted Earth Types, vitamin B12 helps with blood deficient anemia and fatigue. I recommend 500 mcg. of sublingual (under the tongue) B12 with food twice daily.

### White Chestnut (Bach Flower Remedy)

This Bach homeopathic tincture is quite helpful for pensive Earth Types who are overtaxed, overstressed, and physically run down from the resulting mental overstimulation. White Chestnut slows down the endless rotation of worrisome thoughts that wear down the body. Insomnia, obsessive compulsion, worry and anxiety are all candidates for treatment with this tincture. I recommend 3 drops in 3 ounces of water three times per day on an empty stomach.

## ONE PATIENT'S STORY

Janet, whom I would classify as an Earth Type, came to me with a series of immunological problems. She had swollen lymph glands, digestive problems, tooth decay, and bloody gums. She was a former smoker and had a chronic phlegmatic cough. She had sugar cravings and a tendency to over-indulging in sweets, junk foods, and baked goods. She was also consistent-ly overweight by ten to fifteen pounds, and her thyroid was underactive, despite the fact that she was on thyroid medication. Her metabolism was very slow. She also suffered from chronic yeast infections and bloat.

Janet proved to be a very pleasant person, easy to be with. While we talked about her history, I learned that she had a difficult family life and that she was the one who was hold-ing it all together. Clearly, she was in a state of chronic stress which had a lot to do with the role she played in her family.

I suggested that she begin to eat more cooked, warm, and dry foods. I thought it was important for her to have a bit more protein, such as baked fish and poultry, which are con-sidered sweet foods and harmonizing for Earth Types. I also suggested that she have very lean red meat (what is called dieter's lean) a couple of times a week since she had a ten-dency toward deficient levels of vitamin B12 and folic acid. I recommended that she take more sweet, root vegetables such as parsnips, carrots, yams, and acorn squash. Additionally, I told her that pungent vegetables would be good for her, including garlic, onions, leeks, ginger and garlic. I wanted Janet to bake and broil much of her food for the Dry quality baking imparts. Since she needed a bit more Fire, I suggested that she also use some light sautéing with covered pans, and that she limit the variety and volume of her foods.

I put her on the Bach Flower Remedies, White Chestnut, to help relieve her acute anxiety, and Aggrimony, to bind her self-esteem. I also put her on vitamins A and E, diges-tive enzymes to help with bloating and gas, Chromium GTF and glutamine to help reduce her sugar cravings, vitamin C for her bleeding gums, red clover tea for the swollen lymph tissue, and the homeopathic remedy, pulsatilla.

We were able to make a lot of progress with Janet. Now, her gums don't bleed anymore, her lymph glands are normal, her chronic cough has cleared up, she's sleeping well, and she no longer suffers from acute anxiety.

## EARTH BREAKFAST #1

### Muesli

> *1-1/2 cup rolled oats*
> *1-1/2 cups spring water*
> *1 tbsp. apple juice*
> *2 tbsp. rice syrup*
> *1/2 cup dried apples, chopped*
> *1/2 cup dried pears, chopped*
> *1/4 cup currants*
> *2 tbsp. slivered chopped almonds*

In a large bowl combine all of the ingredients. Chill in the refrigerator overnight. Stir well and serve.

## EARTH BREAKFAST #2

### Oatmeal Supreme

> *1 cup oatmeal*
> *3 tbsp. currants*
> *1/2 cup diced apples*
> *3 tbsp. chopped walnuts*
> *1/2 tsp. cinnamon*
> *1/2 tsp. nutmeg*
> *Rice Dream as needed*

Cook the oatmeal as directions call for. Add the apples and cook until soft. Sprinkle on the remaining ingredients.

## EARTH BREAKFAST #3

### Fruity Almond Cream of Rice

*1/4 cup cream of rice*
*1/2 cup organic apple juice*
*1/2 cup spring water*
*2 tsp. rice syrup*
*1 tbsp. diced dried apples*
*1 tbsp. currants*
*1 tbsp. toasted chopped almonds*

In a heavy sauce pan combine the first four ingredients and bring to a boil. Reduce the heat and stir frequently until thick. Serve and sprinkle on the last three ingredients.

## EARTH LUNCH #1

### Rice Pilaf with Almonds

*2 cups cooked brown rice*
*2 tbsp. olive oil*
*1 cup chopped onion*
*3 garlic cloves minced*
*1 tsp. Turmeric*
*2 tbsp. fresh lemon juice*
*2 tbsp. Bragg's Amino Liquid*
*1/2 cup fresh basil, chopped*
*1/2 cup fresh parsley, chopped*
*1 tsp. fresh thyme*
*1/2 cup of sliced almonds*
*Sea salt and pepper to taste*

Sauté onions and garlic in olive oil for 5 minutes. Stir in lemon juice, Bragg's, and turmeric Add herbs and rice and cook on low heat for 5 minutes. Garnish with almonds.

## EARTH LUNCH #2

**Winter Squash Soup**

> *1 large acorn squash*
> *1 tsp. butter*
> *1 medium leek, chopped*
> *1 tbsp. olive oil*
> *1-1/2 chopped sage*
> *Dash of pepper*
> *1/4 tsp. ginger*
> *1/4 tsp. chili powder*
> *1/4 tsp. allspice*
> *1/4 tsp. cinnamon*
> *5 cups natural chicken broth*
> *2 medium Granny Smith apples*

Halve acorn squash and bake for 45 minutes at 375°F, then let cool.

Sauté leeks until soft ,add spices and broth and simmer for 10 minutes. Then add chopped apples and cook until soft. Scoop out acorn squash and add to soup. Let simmer for 5 minutes then place in blender, serve hot.

## EARTH LUNCH #3

**Oat Burger**

> *12 oz. ground turkey*
> *1/2 cup onion*
> *1/2 cup carrots, grated*
> *1/2 cup diced red pepper*
> *3/4 oz. quick oats*
> *Dash ground pepper*
> *1 tbsp. Bragg's Amino Liquid*

Combine all ingredients and press into patties. Broil until cooked through.

## EARTH DINNER #1

**Roasted Turkey Breast**

*2 turkey breasts halved*
*1 tsp. thyme*
*1 tsp. rosemary*
*4 cloves of minced garlic*
*1 tsp. lemon rind*
*1/2 tsp. fresh ground pepper*
*1 cup natural chicken broth*
*1 medium onion*

Place turkey in baking dish. Pour broth over and place wedged onion around turkey. Place remaining ingredients over turkey. Bake at 325°F for 45 minutes.

## EARTH DINNER #2

**Haddock Bake**

*1 pound haddock fillet*
*1 small onion chopped*
*1/4 cup dry white organic wine*
*1 tbsp. butter organic*
*rosemary and thyme to taste*
*1 tbsp. dry mustard*

Combine spices and butter, then spread mixture over filet. Place fillet in parchment bag. Pour in wine and place onions over fillet. Seal the bag and bake at 350°F for 8 minutes on each side or until flaking.

## EARTH DINNER #3

**Root Vegetable Medley**

> *1 cup carrots*
> *1 cup turnips*
> *1 cup parsnips*
> *1 cup yams*
> *1/2 cup onion*
> *2 tsp. of curry powder (or to taste)*
> *1/2 tsp. parsley*
> *1 tbsp. olive oil*
> *Sea salt and pepper to taste*

Dice vegetables. Sauté with olive oil in large skillet until soft. Season with sea salt, pepper and curry. Top with parsley before serving.

NOTE: *Consult with your physician before taking any natural food supplements.*

# CHAPTER 10

# Metal

Metal is as refined as gold, as discerning as a judge, as precise as mathematics, as disciplined as a spiritual master. Seasonally, Metal corresponds to Fall, that time of year when Nature's outward display fades and dies back. The first cold and cutting winds begin to blow intermittently, as the Earth turns away from the Sun and the nights begin to grow long. At this time, Nature is moving inward. Dead leaves and decayed plants fall to the ground to serve as fertilizer for next year's growth. Plants encapsulate their essence into seeds that will sleep away the Winter to awaken in Spring. The bright flowers, plants, and bushes melt back into the Earth from which they came. Squirrels scurry across the ground, gathering stores for Winter. At this time, there is a sense of sadness and loss as all that was born in Spring and grew in Summer dies away once again.

The season corresponding to the Metal Type is the time

to separate the wheat from the chaff; it is the time to take the best from the past and preserve it for the next round of birth and growth. It is a time for culling that which isn't useful any longer and distilling out that which is. Metal is a good time to take stock of resources, sorting through all that has been created in the previous, active seasons. Metal is a time to organize experiences and set goals for the future. It is a time to withdraw from the furious activity that marked Spring and Summer and delve inward to replenish inner resources. It is a time of reminiscing and reflection.

Metal Types, then, take many of their characteristics from the season with which they are linked. As such, they tend to be disciplined, organized, efficient, and structured. They are analytical and critical, often approaching things as though it were their job to report what is wrong with a situation. They have a refined sense of beauty and are idealistic at heart. Metal Types are inwardly focused and have highly developed mental and spiritual natures. They are thoughtful and conscious about what they do, carefully thinking before they act.

Metal Types are conscientious workers who have a strong attraction for order and control. Their excellent ability at scheduling and prioritizing makes them great managers. Because they are so good at dismantling a problem or situation into its component parts, they make great analysts and consultants. They are patient, precise, and detail-oriented. They are goal setters, capable of getting a job done well in a sequenced, orderly fashion. Metal Types have a very refined nature and a reserved demeanor. They tend to be impeccable dressers, with equally impeccable personal habits. They are regal and noble, with a quiet confidence that comes from knowing who they are and what they are doing. They have good boundaries and are not thrown off center by what others think. They are not impulsive and outwardly passionate, but moved by deep convictions based on the way they believe things should be. Metal Types have high principles and are often idealists. They are straight shooters who like predictability, consistency, and routine. If they become imbalanced with an excess of Metal energy, they tend to become obsessive and compulsive. In this case, their natural inclination to be of service to others can turn to self-righteousness and criticism.

While they have a wonderful capacity for discipline, the flip side can be a perfectionism that leads to rigidity. They have a tendency to overwork because they feel comfortable within the structure of a job. Metal Types tend to lack spontaneity in social situations, finding it difficult to be casual and relaxed. Because of this they sometimes appear to be aloof emotionally. It can also be difficult for Metal Types to be intimate with others. It is important for Metal Types to guard against becoming rigid in their thinking and their bodies. It's important for them to learn to go with their intuitive and innovative impulses, so that they don't become robotic in their reliance on the status quo. Metal Types are also inclined to be melancholic. Their Yin nature reflects their tendency to feel sad and withdrawn from the world.

### BASIC CHARACTERISTICS: A SNAPSHOT OF THE METAL TYPE

Metal Types are generally shorter than average with a small to medium sized frame. They have well-defined musculature and tend to be 5-10 pounds underweight. They have dry complexions with thin skin that is often sallow. Typically, they tend to be very blond or platinum haired, with pale blue eyes and cloudy whites. Their appetites tend to be light to moderate, and they are very disciplined eaters. Their elimination vacillates between the two extremes of constipation and diarrhea. Their stamina is generally low, and their endurance is poor. Their typical diseases are of a respiratory nature, and irritable bowel syndrome is common to them. Their positive mental nature is logical, precise and analytical. Their negative mental nature is obsessive and rigid. Emotionally, they can be either courageous and bold or melancholic and depressed. Metal Types have an affinity for order and an aversion to spontaneity. Their basic instinct is to organize and their life's purpose is to implement systems. Metal's positive archetype is the organizer and the negative archetype is the perfectionist.

## METAL AND THE BODY

*The **Metal Power** governs the lung and large intestine.*

The lung is responsible for converting oxygen into Ch'i. Respiration is a very critical life process and impaired lung function results in impaired immune function, rendering the body vulnerable to all kinds of diseases as well as overall weakness, exhaustion and shortness of breath. The lung is responsible for oxygenating the blood and balancing body temperature. The lung (in conjunction with the thyroid) is also responsible for keeping the lymph fluids clean, preventing such symptoms as chronic sinus and inner ear infections.

Additionally, one of the lungs' chief functions is that of hydration, and they work closely with the kidneys to regulate moisture; the lung is thus responsible for hydrating the skin and hair. A healthy lung function will ensure healthy fluid metabolism, whereas unhealthy lungs will lead to swelling and fluid retention, especially in the face and head. Impaired lung function can also lead to urinary retention.

The Chinese say that because the lung openings extend all the way up to the nose, you can learn much about their functioning by observing the breath. An even flow of breath through both nostrils reflects good functioning lungs, whereas blockages and uneven breath indicates impaired function.

## CHARACTERISTIC METAL PROBLEMS

Metal needs to cut — to cut to the point, to cut the bull, to cut through the extraneous to the essential nature of an event, experience, or resource. They are driven to strip things down to an archetypal ideal. When they take this perfectionistic tendency too far, they can become hypocritical, rigid, and dogmatic. Often, if this tendency becomes extreme, Metal Types can become very closed-minded and unyielding in their approach to life. This can result in a rigidity in the body that affects their breathing, their elimination, and almost all of their bodily systems. It is important that this type learn that their way isn't the only way to go. Metal Types need to guard against having too narrow a focus.

Typically, Metal Types suffer from imbalances that result from a tendency to accumulate Dryness and an inability to regulate hydration and lubrication in the body. They tend to suffer from respiratory diseases, and can become run down or depleted by either excessive or repressed emotional sadness.

Depending on the particular time, Metal, like all the types, can suffer either from an excess of high energy or an exhausted, low-energy state. These energetic swings are normal and affect everything in the natural world, including people. When Metal Types are exhausted, they speak softly, or lack a desire to talk at all. Their appetite is generally weak, their energy low, and their spirits lagging. During these times they can suffer from a variety of conditions: dry and itchy hair or skin; dry cough; asthma; fevers; sore throats; swollen tongues; sinus headaches; constipation; dark, scanty urine; tight and stiff muscles; respiratory allergies of a dry nature.

When Metals Types are in a high-energy mode, they can become vulnerable to the following health conditions: bronchitis; cystic fibrosis; lung cancer; breast cancer; rectal/colon cancer; colitis; Chrone's disease; chronic sinus infections; obsessive-compulsive disorder; shortness of breath; incontinence; clammy hands and feet; excessive perspiration; allergies of a wet nature with excessive white or yellow phlegm.

## A HEALING BALANCE FOR METAL

### Pungent: Metal's Medicinal Food Flavor

The pungent food group has a special affinity for all Metal Types. Pungent is an extremely vigorous food energy that is capable of improving circulation, dissolving fatty deposits, distributing moisture to dry lungs and sinuses, and drying up phlegmatic conditions in the lungs. It is also credited with the power to detoxify pathogens and wastes from the intestines, blood and urinary tract.

The pungent food group is said to possess the energy to help clear the lungs of long-standing depression and repressed grief.

### Common examples of the Pungent Food Group:

Carrot, cayenne, cinnamon, currant, bok choy, daikon, garlic, ginger, leek, mustard greens, onion, oregano, parsley, radish, sardine, scallion, turnip, turmeric, white pepper.

## NATURAL MEDICINES FOR METAL

### Antimonium tartaricum *(tartrate of antimony and potash)*

This is a classic natural medicine for any respiratory illness that is accompanied by a non-productive rattling mucous cough, short difficult breath, or a dry, painful cough. Asthma, emphysema, bronchitis, colds and flu are all aided greatly by this medicine especially when there is little expectoration. I recommend it be taken in a 30c potency for up to three weeks—three pellets under the tongue three times per day on an empty stomach.

### Beta I. 3D Glucan

Extracted from the cell walls of Baker's yeast, this powerful immune enhancer has an affinity for supporting immune cell production in the body. Macrophages are immune cells which act like a super powered vacuum cleaner, sweeping through the blood, swallowing up germs, bacteria, viruses and other invaders. It has also demonstrated the ability to protect cells against harmful radiation and free radical damage. In my work, Beta I. 3D Glucan has clearly proven its special effectiveness in helping most Metal Types with lung, lymph, and other general respiratory illnesses, both acute and chronic. I recommend 100 mg. once a day taken on an empty stomach.

### Fenugreek *(Trigonella Foenugraecum)*

This pleasant-tasting tea is superb for all respiratory illnesses which are predominated by a heavy, wet phlegm and congestion. One of the oldest medicinal herbs on the planet, it has been successfully used to treat ulcers, as well as a variety of other inflammatory conditions of the stomach and intestines. For all Metal Types who have either acute or chronic digestive disorders, I recommend 1-3 cups of Fenugreek tea per day.

### Gorse *(Ulex Europaeus)*

Gorse (a homeopathic Bach Flower Remedy) is another natural medicine more attuned for the mind. It is especially appropriate for the Metal Type's mind and heart, as it is intended to help heal grief energy. Designated for sadness, despair, and hopelessness, especially after much long suffering, Gorse is a superb natural medicine for the psyche of most

Metal Types, or, for that matter, almost anyone experiencing those emotions. I recommend three drops dissolved in 3 ounces of water. Sip three times per day on an empty stomach.

### L-Cysteine

This amino acid is a cell membrane stabilizer which serves as a great lung and lymph protector against cigarette smoke and pollution. It has also been shown to stimulate white blood cell immune activity in response to disease. It also breaks down respiratory mucous resulting from infection, allergy and diet. This lung and lymph tonic/cleanser is a superior natural medicine for all Metal Types. I recommend 500 mg. twice a day on an empty stomach.

### Mullein *(Verbascum Thapsus)*

For centuries, this tincture has calmed inflamed and irritated nerves, helping respiratory patients control coughs and coughing spasms. It has the ability to loosen phlegm and help clear it out of the respiratory tract. It also said to both tone and cleanse the respiratory system and is equally medicinal for the tonsils, throat and sinuses; it has even demonstrated the ability to shrink warts and small tumors. I recommend 10-15 drops of Mullein tincture dissolved in 3 ounces of water. Sip three times a day on an empty stomach.

### Myrrh *(Balsamodendron Myrrha)*

Not unlike Mullein, Myrrh is a superb respiratory purgative and tonic. The primary difference is that Myrrh is more of an antiseptic for the mucous membranes of the lung and lymph systems. Myrrh has also been said to give great strength to the stomach and small intestines, but I primarily recommend it as a superb natural medicine for all lung disorders, especially for most Metal Types. I recommend it be taken in tincture form. Dissolve 10-15 drops in 3 ounces of warm or hot water and sip three times a day on an empty stomach.

### Spongia Tosta

This natural homeopathic medicine is indicated for a croupy, wet cough rooted deep in the chest. Good for bronchial catarrh, asthmatic cough which is worse in cold air, and profuse expectoration, this is a superb medicine for most deficient Metal Types. I recommend a 30c potency, taken for three weeks. Dissolve 3 tablets under the tongue three times a day on an empty stomach.

### Borage Oil *(Borago Officinalis)* in capsule form

The prostaglandin action in Borage Oil has been shown to help regulate insulin levels which aids both hypoglycemia and diabetes. It has also demonstrated the ability to help many with multiple sclerosis, prostate inflammation, hormonal imbalances, and obesity. I have witnessed remarkable results when this substance is used therapeutically for hormal problems in both men and women. For Metal Types with general immuno-deficiency problems, this is a valuable aid in treating respiratory problems. Its greatest feature for Metal Types, though, is its anti-inflammatory action which makes it very effective for asthmatic and bronchial inflammations. I recommend 1000 mg. capsules with food three times a day.

### Zinc *(Gluconate)*

Zinc assists with all protein and DNA synthesis in the body. It furthermore supports the lungs with carbon dioxide detoxification and disease resistance. I've found it to be of great help with all respiratory problems, especially where there is significant inflammation accompanied by high level of copper in the body tissue. I recommend 50 mg. of Zinc Gluconate daily taken with food.

## ONE PATIENT'S STORY

Patrick, as I will call him, is an entrepreneur in his mid-50's. He's always dressed to the nines — very neat, prim, and proper.

When I first saw him, Patrick complained of dry hair and skin, tight, stiff muscles, constipation, and a chronic dry cough. As we progressed, I began to see what was most likely, for all intents and purposes, an undiagnosed rheumatoid arthritic condition. This dry, inflammatory response is often described by the Chinese as a Fire condition that dehydrates and inflames the lungs, as well as the joints, muscles, skin, and hair. Thus, it is seen as Fire invading Metal. The lungs and large intestines — Metal's corresponding organs — were struggling to moisturize and hydrate themselves. Metaphorically, they were not able to offset the ravages of Fire.

Since Patrick wouldn't do well with hot and drying foods, I suggested that he refrain from eating pungent foods, such as onions, leeks, scallions, and garlic. He needed foods that would offset Heat and Dryness, while creating coolness and moisture. In keeping with this, I suggested that he use more raw foods (fruits and salads) along with lean proteins, including seafood. I also put Patrick on cod liver oil to hydrate his dry skin and flax oil for his bowels. I suggested that he take the homeopathic remedy, Antimonium, for his dry respiratory, allergy-type problems. I did extensive testing on him for allergies to determine what foods he was sensitive to, and suggested that he eliminate those foods.

Patrick's recovery was dramatic and he is now a rare visitor.

## ANOTHER PATIENT'S STORY

The following story is a first-person account in the patient's own words.

*"I'd been seeing a number of dermatologists for at least ten, or closer to 15 years. The problem was constant itching and dry, peeling skin on my hands and face. I would itch and I'd scratch it and it would bleed. The dermatologists called it eczema. I finally found one doctor I thought I was satisfied with, and I stayed with him for about five years. He'd give me medicine, and it would clear up then just come back again. Finally, he gave up and sent me to a doctor in Boston who sent me to another doctor who was supposedly an expert. I tried a bunch of treatments with him — ultraviolet light and various ointments and prescription drugs; finally he just said he didn't know what it was.*

*Then a friend of mine where I used to work recommended Dr. Mincolla and I went down and saw him and what a difference! Almost immediately. Even just from talking to him I felt a lot better. He looked me over and told me to stay away from red meat and dairy products. He found a few fruits I should stay away from most of the time — I could have them once in a while just like I could have a hamburger every three months or so; that isn't going to bother me. I started using rice milk on cereal, instead of regular milk and there's an ice cream made out of rice I can use, too, if I want. He also put me on a bunch of herbs and vitamins I can't even pronounce. Every time I left his office he would say, "Hey this is no real problem." And this is after 15 years of other doctors!*

*Almost immediately I got relief, and that was it. It was amazing. Right now, my hands and face are totally clear, no more itching and scratching. I've been seeing Dr. Mincolla a couple times a year for about three years and everybody's happy — I mean the rest of my family. It had been kind of miserable for them, too.*

*So, diet and vitamins and paying attention to what he recommended is what did it. I'm very satisfied. Couldn't be happier."*

## METAL BREAKFAST #1

### Black Currant and Ginger Pears

*5-6 firm ripe pears, peeled and sliced thin*
*1-1/2 cup black currant juice*
*2 tsp. finely ch. ginger root*
*2 tbs. arrowroot*
*1/4 cup cold water*

Add juice, ginger and pears to saucepan. Boil and simmer 15 min., or until soft. Dilute arrowroot in water. Add to pears and stir until thick. Serve.

## METAL BREAKFAST #2

### Cinnamon Rice Pudding with Currants

*1 cup rice milk*
*1/4-1/3 cup brown rice syrup*
*1/2 tsp. ground cinnamon or 2 cinnamon sticks*
*1 tsp. vanilla or maple extract*
*2 cups cooked short-grain brown rice*
*1/3-1/2 cup currants*

Preheat oven to 350°F. Blend rice milk and rice syrup in blender. Add cinnamon and vanilla and blend again. Combine with cooked rice and add currants. Bake in 9x13 dish for 45 min.

## METAL BREAKFAST #3

### Eggless Omelet

*1 lb. firm tofu*
*1 cup soy or rice milk*
*1 scallion, finely chopped  2 tbsp. olive oil*
*1/2 cup bok choy, sliced thin*

*1 leek, sliced thin*
*1/2 med. onion, sliced thin*
*1/2 pepper, sliced thin*
*2 garlic cloves, pressed*
*1 cup mustard greens*
*Pepper to taste*
*Fresh parsley for garnish*

Heat oven to 400°F. Drain tofu and crumble. Place tofu, soy or rice milk in blender and blend until smooth. Stir in scallion. Place in two pie plates and bake for 35 min. Meanwhile, heat 1 tbsp. oil in skillet. Add remaining ingredients and cook until tender. Add pepper and parsley to taste. Cover omelet with vegetable topping.

## METAL LUNCH #1

### Boston Baked Navy Beans

*2 cup pre-soaked navy beans*
*5 cup water*
*3/4 med. onion, chopped*
*3 tbsp. Bragg's Amino Liquid*
*1 tbsp. olive oil*
*1-2 tsp. dry mustard*
*1 tsp. ground ginger*
*1/2 tsp. garlic powder*
*1/2 cup rice syrup*
*1/2 cup currants (optional)*

Place beans and water in saucepan and cook on low heat for 45 min. (save cooking liquid). Preheat oven to 350°F. In dish or bean pot, mix beans, onions, Bragg, oil and currants. In a separate bowl, mix rice syrup and spices and 2 cups of liquid from beans or water. Add to beans in pot. Bake covered for 1–3 hours. Add water if mixture gets too dry.

## METAL LUNCH #2

### Turkey Burgers or Meatballs over Rice

*1/2 tsp. basil, tarragon, celery seed, sage, oregano,*
*thyme, marjoram (or any combination)*
*1/4 tsp. white pepper, cayenne or chili pepper,*
*garlic powder, ground ginger*
*1 tbsp. fresh parsley*
*1/4 cup onion, chopped fine*
*2 tbsp. brown rice or oat flour*
*1 lb. ground turkey breast*
*Paprika*

Mix spices (except paprika) with flour and then with turkey. Form into burger or meatball shape and sprinkle paprika on top. Bake in 400°F oven for 15–20 min. Serve over brown rice.

### Creamy Brown Gravy

*2 tbsp. brown rice flour*
*2 tbsp. canola oil*
*1/3-2/3 cup vegetable or chicken broth*
*1 tbsp. onion powder*
*1 tsp. basil*
*1/2 tsp. garlic powder*
*1/4 tsp. oregano*
*1 tsp. dried parsley*

Heat oil on med. and stir in flour until smooth. Slowly stir in broth and seasoning and cook, stirring until thick or desired consistency.

## METAL LUNCH #3

### Cauliflower Bisque

*1 tsp. olive oil*
*4 cups water or vegetable broth*
*1/2 cup sliced onions*
*1/2 cup sliced leeks*
*1 med. cauliflower, florets*
*1 cup soy milk*
*1/2 cup soy flour*
*2 garlic cloves*
*Bragg's Amino Liquid*
*1/8 tsp. pepper*
*1 tbsp. fresh or 2 tsp. dried dill*
*toasted walnuts*

Heat oil and cook onion 10 min. Add garlic and cook 1 more minute. Add broth, cauliflower, soy milk, pepper and simmer for 30-45 minutes. Blend until creamy. Sprinkle with toasted walnuts and dill.

## METAL DINNER #1

### Black Bean Salad

> *2 cups black beans*
> *1 cup diced tomatoes*
> *1-1/2 cup diced Bell Peppers*
> *(red, yellow or green pepper mixture)*
> *1 tbsp. fresh chopped Cilantro*
> *1 tsp. ground cumin*
> *1 tsp. ground coriander*
> *1 tsp. cayenne pepper*
> *1 tbsp. lime juice or lemon juice*
> *2 tbps. olive oil*
> *1 cup brown rice*

In small bowl combine, cilantro, cumin, coriander, cayenne, lemon or lime juice and olive oil. Stir in beans, tomatoes, peppers and rice. Refrigerate until ready to serve.

## METAL DINNER #2

### Ginger Chicken

> *2 tsp. Bragg's Amino Liquid*
> *1 tsp. grated fresh ginger root*
> *1 garlic clove, minced*
> *(4) 4 oz. skinless chicken breasts*

In small dish combine Bragg's, ginger and garlic. Add chicken and marinate for 3 hours. Broil on each side for 8-10 minutes.

## METAL DINNER #3

**Fish Stew**

> *1/2 lb. fresh haddock, flounder or scrod*
> *1 lb. tofu cut in 1" cubes*
> *4 slices ginger root*
> *1 tsp. Bragg's Amino Liquid*
> *1 stalk celery*
> *2 scallions*
> *1 cup vegetable or chicken broth*
> *2 tbsp. chopped fresh parsley, dill, or basil*
> *2 tbsp. coriander*

Place all but parsley and coriander in pot and cover. Cook 30 min., or until fish flakes with a fork. Garnish with parsley and coriander.

NOTE: *Consult with your physician before taking any natural food supplements.*

# CHAPTER 11

# Water

Water is as deep as the ocean, as penetrating as the cold, as yielding as air, as pervasive as night. Water is linked with Winter, the most Yin, or inactive, season of the year. At this time, Nature has turned inward to regenerate itself in preparation for the new, active cycle that will come with Spring. It is as though the Earth is pregnant with a million gestating life forms sheltered in the deep womb of Nature. Water is a quiet time of death and regeneration when the miracle of life is being born beneath the surface of the phenomenal world. With Water, Nature has reached its most extreme point of inwardly-focused being. Water's nature is to yield, and through its ability to yield it is capable of transforming that which appears to be unmoveable, just as a canyon can be created by the gentle meander of a river across rock. The subtle action of water belies its incredible power.

Water Types, then, are the least physically, outwardly

active of the Five Types. They are the most introspective, the most sensitive, the most mentally and spiritually developed. This, however, does not mean that they are not strong. Their strength lies in their connection with the inner worlds and the source of all being. Frequently Water Types are deep, brilliant thinkers. They are serious and perceptive, original and doggedly determined to think things through. They are enigmatic and unusual, dancing to the beat of a different drummer. Water Types are interested in what lies beneath the surface. They are the philosophers who want to know why we exist, what we are, where we come from, and where we are going. It is their function to extract the deep meaning behind appearances.

Although Water Types are deeply emotional, they aren't good at small talk and don't do well in large social situations. Water Types tend to be loners who frequently have a hard time connecting with the outside world while at the same time they are acutely aware of their internal connection to the universe. If you do find a Water Type at a party, she will not be the center of a large and laughing crowd like the Fire Type, but sitting in one spot deep in conversation with another. Water Types are thinkers rather than doers. They are visionaries who have unusual, far-out thoughts. They are very affected by the unconscious and the realm of dreams and intuitions. Water Types tend to artistic and scholarly pursuits, often making art themselves. Frequently, they are wise beyond their years.

Water Types are voracious readers, and typically highly educated, frequently self-taught. They are natural teachers, who teach what they learn. It is very important for Water Types to maintain contact with others so that they don't get isolated and frozen in their own little world, just as water turns to ice. If this extreme situation evolves, the Water Type can become very fearful, feeling lost and alone. Physically, this can manifest as frailty, low-energy and poor endurance. When they go too far in this direction, they can become very fearful, despondent, paranoid, and suspicious. On the other hand, when they are in a period of positive flow (their energy is flowing well) their creativity abounds. They can be way ahead of others with their brilliance at physics or art or history. When they are not in a positive flow, their thoughts can get very ungrounded and cross over into the realm of strange, fragmented thinking.

Because of Water's tendency to be withdrawn, they often find it hard to maintain a positive frame of mind and become easily discouraged. At these times, they can lose touch with the world and with their own strength and self-sufficiency. At such times, they lose concentration and have a hard time distinguishing between reality and unreality. This can overburden their immune systems, which often results in sudden and dramatic illness. More than any other Type, Water Types must be diligent about taking care of themselves and remaining grounded in the material world. It is important for them to get plenty of quality rest and sleep to recharge themselves. Although it often seems as if they are hanging onto the physical world by a thin thread, they have a surprising resilience due to their spiritual strength which frequently carries them through.

## BASIC CHARACTERISTICS: A SNAPSHOT OF THE WATER TYPE

Water Types tend to be on the short side, with thin, wiry frames and little muscular definition. Their weight is usually 10 pounds or more under the average. Their skin tends to be pale and thin, and they often have dark circles under their eyes. Their thin hair is characteristically jet black, turning, perhaps prematurely, to salt and pepper as they age. The eyes of Water Types are typically deep blue, with very white irises. Their appetites range from low to very low. Their elimination is frequently loose, their stamina low, and their physical endurance poor. Their pulses are slow and shallow at approximately 40-50 beats per minute. The most characteristic diseases of the Water Type are genito-urinary, hormonal, and blood deficiencies. Their positive mental nature is cautious and conservative, and their negative mental nature is stagnant. Emotionally, they can range from calm and peaceful to fearful and disassociated. They have an affinity for solitude and an aversion to exposure. Their basic instinct is to yield and their life's purpose is to teach. Water's positive archetype is the genius and negative archetype is the recluse.

## WATER AND THE BODY

*The Water Type governs the kidney and bladder.*

The kidneys are responsible for reproduction, growth, development, and the balancing of fluids. It is thought that our prenatal essence, or hereditary influences, are stored in the kidneys. The Chinese called this essence Jing, and believed it to be largely responsible for our constitutional strength. The kidneys are thought to be the gateway to all vitality. The kidney is also responsible for refining the essence we extract from food, specifically ribonucleic acid, or protein.

Kidney impairment can result in sexual disorders, problems with growth, learning disabilities, premature ejaculation, impotence and urinary infections. In children, the kidneys are responsible for the development of good bone marrow, which is vital to the production of blood. If the marrow is impaired, the brain, the bones and the spinal cord all suffer. These problems can result in serious immune problems, tinnitus, blurred vision, lower back pains, impaired thinking.

On the upper portion of the kidneys sit the adrenal glands, which are responsible for Heat in the body. Because of this, the Chinese call them the lakes of fire. The lower kidney is the fluid balancer of the body, and is called the lakes of water, or the drainage ditch. The kidneys open up into the ears and manifest in the hair. Hearing problems indicate a deficient kidney function. Loss of hair, poor hair quality, and premature graying can reflect poor kidney function. Excess fear stores in the kidneys. Conversely, poor kidney function will show itself as fear, weakness, timidity, and hypersensitivity.

### CHARACTERISTIC WATER PROBLEMS

It is Water's nature to withdraw from the outside world and delve inward. In keeping with this, their mind-body energy tends to be withdrawn and less physically vital than that of the other types. While their emotions and mental activity run deep, their stamina runs low. They also tend toward overly active nervous systems. Depending on the particular time, Water, like all the Types, can suffer either from an excess of high-energy or an exhausted, low-energy state. These energetic swings are normal and affect everything in the natural world, including people.

When Water Types are experiencing a period of high energy they can become vulnerable to a range of conditions, including the following: kidney and bladder stones; nephritis; chronic bladder problems; kidney infections; bone tumors; gum disease; insomnia; deviant sexual behavior; impotence; hypertension; vision headaches; deficient perspiration and urine; hardening of the arteries; hypersensitive nervous reflex systems; uterine and prostrate cancer; bone cancer; osteoporosis; osteoarthritis; super erratic behavior.

When, on the other hand, this Type is experiencing an exhausted, low-energy period they can become vulnerable to

another range of conditions such as: poor stamina; weak or
stiff lower spine; cold extremities; osteoporosis; lack of stamina; disc degeneration; infertility; frigidity; impotence;
insecurity; anxiety; excessive fears and in extreme cases, ago-
raphobia, or the fear of going out into the world.

## A HEALING BALANCE FOR WATER

### Salty: Water's Primary Medicinal Food Flavor

The salty food group is able to moisten and lubricate the
lungs and intestines. It is also credited with the power to soft-
en and dissolve lumps, tumors and nodes. Salt foods are
especially suited to the sick and inactive types, it is considered
the primary food medicine for all Water types. Salty foods are
also credited with the power to neutralize anxiety, unfocused
thinking and poor concentration.★

### Common examples of the Salty Food Group:

Arame, bibb lettuce, bluefish, chestnuts, collard greens,
dulse, earth salt, grapes, hijiki, kelp, kombu, navy beans, nori,
olive, parsley, pinto beans, red clover, sea salt, sorrel, spinach,
Swiss chard.

## NATURAL MEDICINES FOR WATER EXCESS

### Cranberry *(juice)*

Cranberries possess chemical components that shield
human urinary tract cells from bacteria. Recent research sug-

---

★The salty food group should be strictly avoided by all those who are overweight or have high
blood pressure or diseases of the blood. All Fire and Wood types should also strictly avoid the salty
food group.

gests they have the ability to reduce the risk of bladder and kidney infection by as much 40%! Considering that it takes 147 dried extract capsules to equal one 8-ounce glass of juice, I recommend 3-5 glasses of cranberry juice per week for those Water Types who are prone to kidney or bladder infections. I suggest you buy the more wholesome brands that are less sugary, and blended with apple or some other less tart juice.

### Eupatorium parpureum *(homeopathic Queen of the Meadow)*

This age-old remedy is most helpful with deep, dull kidney pain, lower back pain, kidney or bladder infections, enlarged prostate, as well as impotence and sterility. It is clearly an ideal natural medicine for deplete Water Types. I recommend the tablets in a 30c potency, taken for three weeks. Three tablets dissolved under the tongue three times a day on an empty stomach.

### Mimulus Guttatus *(Bach Flower Remedy)*

This tincture is a superb medicine for the chronic known fears and apprehensions which typically haunt the Water Type. It is also quite helpful for timidity, lack of self esteem and self-assuredness. I recommend 3 drops in 3 ounces of water three times per day on an empty stomach, taken as needed indefinitely.

### Multi-Enzymes *(with Betaine HCL and Ox Bile)*

Water types classically have great difficulty filtering proteins and calciums from the diet. This places great stress on the kidneys. The multi-enzymes containing HCL are especially designed to help in these areas of digestion, taking the burden off the kidneys. I recommend that one tablet be taken at meal time unless there is a history of stomach ulcers, and that usage be discontinued if there is a burning sensation in the stomach. Never take these with light meals or a snack.

### Raw Kidney *(Freeze dried bovine tablets)*

These bio-regulators are very powerful kidney tonics which were first popularized in the Classic European Health Spas in the 1930's. Movie stars and chiefs of state would travel around the world for injections of these raw bovine tissues. Nowadays, they are in the form of freeze dried pills available at your neighborhood health food stores. I recommend one 500 mg. tablet per day taken with food for up to one month at a time.

### Rhemmannia *(Glutinosa)*

This classic Chinese medicinal herb has been used as a kidney tonic for centuries. The unprocessed root, or "sangday" as the Chines call it, is considered the most superior of all herbs as an alkalizer of the blood, and a fortifier of the kidneys. It is also quite useful in treating menstrual irregularities and infertility. I recommend two 1,000 mg. capsules taken every day on an empty stomach.

### Uva Ursi *(Anctostaphylos)* also known as BearBerry

This is useful for cystitis, nephritis, and urethritis. It is a reliable diuretic, astringent, and has urinary antiseptic properties. I recommend two 1000 mg. capsules daily on an empty stomach.

### Vitamin A *(Retinol)*

Vitamin A has long proven its usefulness for Water Types. It is responsible for sperm production, egg development, and mucous membrane formation. As far back as the 1960's, Adelle Davis wrote about the great importance of Vitamin A as an agent to keep the kidneys clear of arterial protein and calcium plaques. I recommend 10,000 units per day.

### Vitamin B2 *(Riboflavin)*

Not unlike Vitamin A, Vitamin B2 is an antagonist to excess boron (a mineral) and calcium deposits in the kidneys. Like Vitamin A, B2 keeps sluggish, weak kidneys clean and clear. I recommend 50 mg. with food twice a day.

### Zinc

This remains the premier fertility supplement. Among its many functions, it helps with sterility, impotence, prostate inflammation and kidney disease. Zinc is an essential core nutrient for all Water Types. I recommend 25mg. per day with food.

### ONE PATIENT'S STORY

Andrew, as I will call him, first came to me three years ago in his mid-30's. He is approximately 5'8" (shorter than average by today's standards) and small-boned. Andrew was thin at the time of our first meeting, and yet his abdomen was distended; he had a pot belly from a build-up of fluid in his lower intestines. Andrew had a frail quality to him; his voice was soft and his presence was light, as opposed to solid or grounded or earthy. His hair had begun to thin when he was in his 20's, and he had a receding hairline. His eyes were very translucent blue like water, very attractive, and the whites were very white. At the time of our meeting, his skin had a bleached look about it.

Andrew complained about a variety of ailments, including frequent achiness in his Achilles tendon and heels, lower back pain, frequent cystitis, and chronic urinary problems. He had difficulty sustaining an erection and experienced premature ejaculation, which were very damaging to his male psyche. His overall stamina was low and he had difficulty performing tasks, was often ill, and frequently missed work. After compiling a history on Andrew, I determined that he was primarily a Water Constitutional Type in a state of low-energy.

Andrew was very interested in using natural therapies to overcome his problems. I recommended that he discontinue the use of raw foods and fruits, even in summer. I suggested that he eat more root vegetables, such as carrots, turnips, and parsnips. I also suggested that he increase his use of very lean, (top round, 95% fat-free) red meat to several times per week. He needed the B12, iron, and folic acid from meat to bind him together and strengthen him—to bring some Yang energy to his overly Yin state. I recommended that he use pungent spices, such as onion powder, garlic, cayenne, and turmeric. I told him to drink two cups of wild Siberian ginseng tea every day — a powerful Yang tonic. I suggested that he sauté much of his food in oil in a covered pan to increase its Yang properties.

I put Andrew on two tablespoons per day of emulsified fish oil, a potent source of Omega-3 essential fatty acids. He also began taking 10,000 units of Vitamin A and two-250 mg. raw kidney tablets daily, along with a multi-enzyme with each of his three meals to help him digest his food. Typically, Water Types don't digest protein very well although they need more of it than other Constitutional Types. I also suggested that Andrew begin practicing Ch'i Gung exercises, which he did.

Andrew and I talked quite a bit about his childhood years, and the fearful environment in which he had lived. We used visualization exercises in many sessions in order to create clear imagery of self-esteem and self-empowerment, which worked well for him.

Andrew made all of these changes and about six months after he first came to me, he began to show marked improvement in many of his problem areas. Now, almost all of his symptoms are gone. He has to be quite strict with his diet; he can't indulge in sugars, fruit juices, fruits, or dairy products very much at all. His sexual life is normal and he rarely misses work anymore. His stamina is better, his urinary tract infections are all cleared up, and his low back pain is all but gone. He is very pleased with his improvement, and I now see him only once a year for check-ups.

### WATER BREAKFAST #1

**Brown Rice Muffins**

> *2 cups brown rice flour*
> *1/2 cup of ground almonds*
> *Egg substitute equiv. to one egg*
> *1/4 cup honey*
> *1 tsp. vanilla extract*
> *1 cup vanilla soy milk*
> *2 tbsp. vegetable oil*

Combine all of the dry ingredients. Combine all of the wet ingredients. Combine both mixtures into a large bowl. Fill muffin tin 3/4 of the way and bake for 25 to 30 minutes at 350°F.

### WATER BREAKFAST #2

**French Toast**

> *1 loaf of yeast free sourdough bread*
> *1 cup of vanilla soy milk*
> *2 eggs or egg substitute*
> *1 tsp. of almond extract*
> *1/2 tsp. cinnamon, nutmeg and allspice*

Combine the last four ingredients and mix well in a large bowl. Slice the bread and dip into the egg mixture. Place in a baking dish and bake for 20 to 30 minutes at 350°F. Flip them after 10 to 15 min.

## WATER BREAKFAST #3

Oat Flour Scones

> *1-1/2 cups oat flour*
> *3 tsp. baking powder*
> *4 tsp. rice syrup*
> *4 tbsp. dairy free sour cream*
> *4 tsp. vegetable oil*
> *2 eggs or egg substitute*

Mix all the dry ingredients together. Then mix all the liquid ingredients together. Combine both mixtures and blend well. Drop rounded tbsp of the batter onto a greased baking sheet. Bake for 15 min. at 350°F or until lightly brown.

## WATER LUNCH #1

Salmon Kebobs

> *12 oz. Salmon*
> *2 tbsp. water*
> *2 tbsp. Bragg's Amino Liquid*
> *1 tbsp. lemon juice*
> *1 tsp. minced onion*
> *1 tsp. minced garlic clove*
> *1/2 tsp. pepper*
> *1/2 tsp. basil*
> *1 medium zucchini, sliced 1 medium onion*

Marinate salmon in the first 7 ingredients for two hours. Place salmon, onion and zucchini on skewers and grill.

## WATER LUNCH #2

### Rosemary Roasted Potatoes

*1lb of Red Bliss potatoes*
*1 tbsp. fresh rosemary*
*3 cloves of garlic*
*2 tbsp. olive oil*
*1 tbsp. of butter*
*Salt and pepper to taste*

Sauté garlic in olive oil and butter with the rosemary until garlic is soft.

Dice potatoes and add to the oil and rosemary mixture in the skillet for approx. 10 minutes. Transfer all the ingredients to a baking dish and bake in preheated oven for 40 minutes at 350°F.

## WATER LUNCH #3

### Lemon Chicken

*1 cup natural chicken broth*
*2 tbsp. lemon juice*
*2 skinned 8 oz. chicken breasts*
*2 tsp. olive oil*
*1/2 tsp. thyme*
*1/2 tsp. rosemary*
*1/2 tsp. tarragon*
*Dash pepper and garlic powder*

Pour broth and lemon juice into small baking dish. Rub each chicken breast with oil and place in dish. Sprinkle with seasonings and bake at 350°F.

## WATER DINNER #1

### Roasted Chicken Breast

> *1 roasting chicken*
> *2 tbsp. fresh rosemary*
> *10 cloves of garlic*
> *2 medium onions*
> *2 tsp. olive oil*

Preheat oven at 450°F, place garlic and rosemary under the skin of breasts and drumsticks. Brush onions with olive oil and arrange around chicken. Cook at 450°F for 30 minutes then at 350°F for 1 hour and 15 minutes. Baste frequently, insert meat thermometer prior to placing in the oven. Remove when it registers at 180°F.

## WATER DINNER #2

### Lamb Kebobs

> *12 oz. lamb*
> *2 tbsp. water*
> *2 tbsp. Bragg's Amino Liquid*
> *1/2 cup of pineapple juice*
> *1 tsp. onion*
> *1 garlic clove*
> *1/2 cup pineapple cubes*
> *1/2 cup red peppers/green peppers cubed*

Marinate lamb in water, Bragg's, pineapple juice, onion and garlic. Place lamb and last two ingredients on skewers and grill until cooked through.

## WATER DINNER #3

**Grilled Veal Dinner**

> *1 tsp. olive oil*
> *1 pound veal scaloppini*
> *1/4 tsp. salt*
> *1/4 tsp. pepper*

Brush oil over veal ,and sprinkle with salt and pepper. Cook 2 minutes on each side or until done. Arrange veal on top of mashed sweet potatoes and butternut squash.

**Mashed Sweet Potatoes and Butternut Squash**

> *2 medium sweet potatoes*
> *1 medium butternut squash*
> *1/2 tsp. sea salt*
> *1/2 tsp. pepper*
> *1/2 tsp. cinnamon*
> *1/2 tsp. nutmeg*
> *1/2 tsp. allspice*
> *1/2 tsp. ginger*
> *1 tbsp. fresh lemon juice*
> *2 tbsp. rice syrup*

Preheat oven 350°F. Put the butternut squash halves upside down on a cookie sheet. Place in oven with the sweet potatoes, until both are soft, about 45 min., then let cool. Scoop out the insides of the squash and potatoes. Mash together with the remaining ingredients.

NOTE: *Consult with your physician before taking any natural food supplements.*

# CHAPTER 12

# Five Simple
# Ta'i Ch'i Exercises

I learned the following Ta'i Ch'i exercises from my dear friend, Master Tom Tam. Tom's loving guidance has not only enhanced my work, but also my life.

Ta'i Ch'i can be thought of as a moving meditation in that it is a form of physical exercise that promotes a deep, meditative relaxation in both the body and the mind. This is accomplished through various mind-body mechanisms that trigger the release of biochemicals into the body when the mind is relaxed. Such chemicals, including an array of neuropeptides and immune enhancers such as interferon, have a decidedly healing effect on the mind-body. In simple terms, Ta'i Ch'i balances the body's life-force energy, or Ch'i, which results in better health and well-being.

Ta'i Ch'i promotes flexibility and strength, both physically and mentally. It is a gentle form of exercise that can be practiced by people of any age. Ta'i Ch'i helps to rebuild both the spirit and the body. Diligent practice will impart a grate-fulness to the mind and body, while improving the health in a variety of ways including better digestion, better breathing, increased lung function, lower blood pressure, and increased blood circulation.

Ultimately, Ta'i Ch'i improves overall health by stimulat-ing a strong flow of Ch'i throughout the mind–body.

Note: Should you become uncomfortable while practic-ing these positions, don't become alarmed. It is normal for you to feel some shaking or perhaps to feel hot or cold. If you become nauseous or dizzy, you may find that you are hungry or tired. If this is the case, stop and drink some hot tea, or eat something light and relax a while before continuing with the exercises. Do not expose yourself to cold or direct wind while practicing, as this may make you vulnerable to a cold or flu attack as a result of energetic weakness.

It is important that beginners make no effort to breath in any special way; the breath should be natural and effortless. During practice, you may keep your eyes open or closed, whichever way feels most comfortable for you.

## EXERCISE 1:
## WOO-CH'I...BEFORE THE BEGINNING

Stand with your feet shoulder width apart. Let your arms hang from your shoulders loosely, hands at at your sides, with the palms facing back. Your hands should be open and relaxed, not stretched or straightened tensely. Bend your knees slightly as if you were about to sit on a tall stool. (The slight bend of the knees will cause your hips to tilt forward, straightening the inward curve in the small of your back.) Keep your head erect, tilted slightly forward as though it were suspended on a string attached to its center. Touch the tip of your tongue to the palate where the teeth and gums meet. This connection

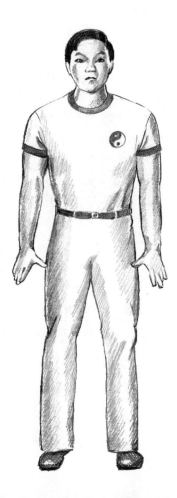

between the tongue and palate completes an energy circuit that helps with the smooth flow of Ch'i. Your weight should be evenly distributed between your toes and heels.

Your eyes can be either open or closed. Some people feel dizzy with their eyes closed. If this occurs, just open your eyes and the sensation should pass within five to ten minutes. Breathe naturally through the nose. Relax your entire body. Let the weight of your body sink into the floor. You may visualize a waterfall flowing through your body. The water enters through the top of your head, slowly washing the tension from every muscle and organ of your body as it flows down toward your toes. After the water soothes your feet, imagine it disappearing into the ground.

As you relax, your breathing will begin to calm and you will start to feel more centered and grounded. Initially, you may feel nothing, or perhaps a tingling or feeling of heat in the palms or elsewhere in the body. This is a normal reaction. It is the natural feeling of Ch'i beginning to move in the body. When you feel Ch'i, refrain from becoming overly excited or frightened; just let the feeling take its course.

This stance is called Wu Ch'i, or Ma Bu. Through the stillness of the body, practitioners can feel the internal movement of Ch'i. This state of being is called "outside silence and inside vibration." You can stand in this posture for five to ten minutes or longer if you enjoy the movement. Do not underestimate the value or importance of this stance because there is no outward movement. Practicing it will bring mental and physical benefits in a short period of time. It brings relaxation and renewed energy.

### EXERCISE 2:
### THE BEGINNING OF TA'I CH'I

Begin by gently turning the hands palms up and raising them, slowly and softly, to shoulder height. Allow the shoulder joint to lift the upper arm, the elbow, the forearm, the wrist, and the hand. When your hands reach shoulder height, your palms should be facing upward toward the sky, as though holding Ch'i from the universe.

Your arms will be extended and your elbows bent (not locked). Gauge the extension of your arms so that shoulders, elbow, and wrists are comfortable. At their highest point, the wrists and elbows should be equidistant from the ground. The arms should be slightly bent and the elbows lower than the wrists and shoulders. Allow gravity to pull the elbows down into a comfortable position. This movement should be gentle, slow, and soft. There should be no resistance in the arms and shoulders. When resistance is low and your position is relaxed, bio-electricity moves more freely. It is not uncommon for people to experience shaking, tingling, or heat in the hands and body when doing this movement. This is a natural consequence of Ch'i, and the release of habitual tension.

According to Chinese medical philosophy, there are six meridian pathways along each arm. Three originate in the torso and upper arm and run all the way to the tip of the fingers, and three originate at the tip of the fingers and run back to the torso and head. When Ch'i moves, different meridians have different reactions.

When the arms are raised to shoulder height, turn your hands over softly, so that your palms are perpendicular with the ground. Gently lower your arms, tilting your hands slightly as your arms get closer to your waist. Use the same speed in lowering your arms as you did in raising them. When your hands are in the Wu Ch'i position, begin the movement again. Raise and lower the hands six times, or in multiple sets of six, as long as you remain comfortable doing so. If you begin to feel uncomfortable (nauseous or dizzy) return to the starting position and relax.

Now that you understand the mechanics of the exercises, think about the meaning. When the palms raise and face upward, you are gathering energy from the sky or heaven. This

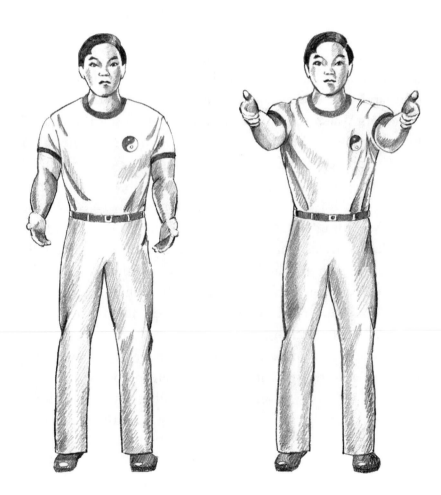

is Yang energy. When the hands reach shoulder level and the palms turn down toward the ground, it is the end of Yang energy, and the start of gathering Yin energy from the Earth. It is important that each time the Yin movement is done, the hands return to the Wu Ch'i beginning posture.

Again, do not be alarmed if your body shakes or heats up. It is eliminating excessive tension in order to return to a balanced state. Move, shake, release the Heat, the Cold, the Wind, the Dampness, and after it is gone, you will feel much better.

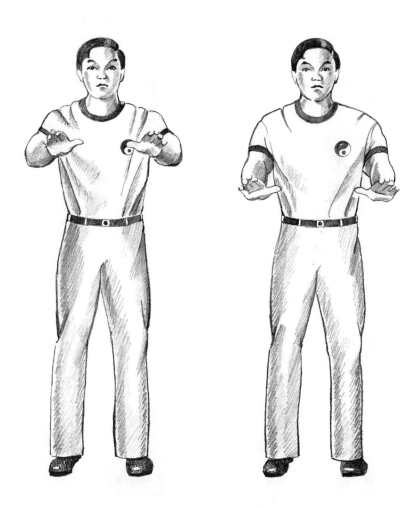

## EXERCISE 3: BRINGING THE CH'I DOWN TO THE DANTIEN

Raise the right hand up to the level of the head, with the palm perpendicular to the front of the body. Again, allow the shoulder joint to lift the upper arm, elbow, forearm, wrist, and hand in that order. Turn the palm toward the body and lower it to your abdomen, keeping your hand six to eight inches from your body. This is where the Dantien is located, or the "storage tank" for the body's internal energy. It is approximately three inches below the navel and one to two inches below the surface of the skin. There are differing opinions concerning the preciselocation of the Dantien, but everyone agrees that it is located in the abdominal area.

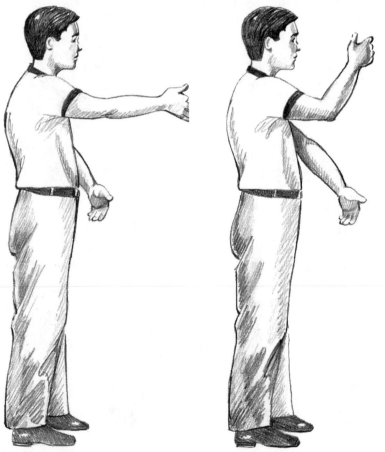

Now, raise the left hand slowly up to the level of the head, keeping the palm perpendicular to the front of the body. Remember that the shoulder lifts the rest of the arm. Turn the palm toward the body and lower it to the Dantien. Continue to alternate hands until each hand has brought the energy to the Dantien six times.

Many beginners have a difficult time coordinating the movement of two hands at the same time. If you find this routine difficult, you can try moving first one hand and then the other. Or you can try imagining that you are climbing a rope or a pole. Remember, while one hand is going up the other hand is going down, and the two hands move in front of you in a circular motion.

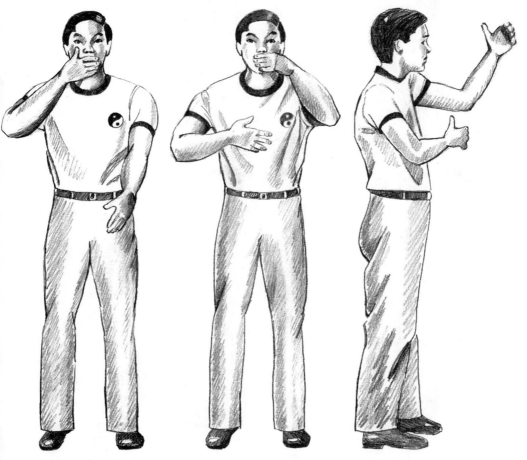

## EXERCISE 4:
## LEADING THE CH'I TO THE PALM

Raise the left arm to shoulder height with the palm facing the sky. The wrist is no higher than the shoulder, and the elbow is slightly bent. Place the palm of the right hand two to four inches above the heart. Then, starting at the left shoulder, gently move the right hand down the length of the left arm. At the same time, the left elbow bends and lowers, pulling the left palm back. Keep a two- to four-inch distance between the

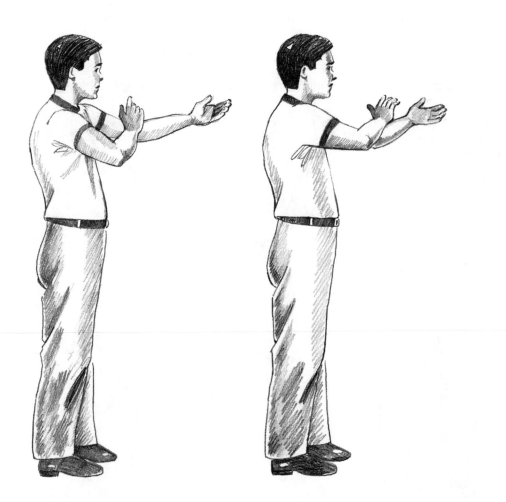

right palm and the left arm as the right palm moves down the left arm. The left palm moves to the left side of the body, finishing the movement at the waist. The palm still faces the sky. The right palm extends forward, always at shoulder height. The elbow is not locked when the right arm is extended beyond the finger tips of the left hand. The right arm extends, finishing the movement with the palm facing the Earth, the wrist in line with, and no higher than the right shoulder, with elbows slightly bent.

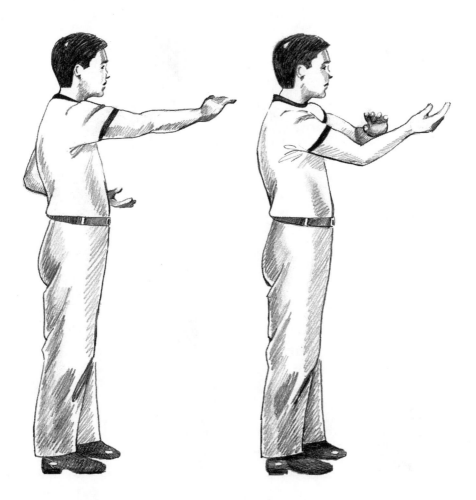

Next, rotate the wrist of the right hand so that the palm faces the sky. Place the left palm two to four inches above the heart. Gently move the left hand toward the right shoulder and down the length of the right arm as the right elbow bends and lowers, pulling the palm back. Now, rotate the wrist of the left hand so the palm faces the sky.

This movement makes people feel calm and relaxed because the pericardium meridian in Chinese medicine helps to regulate emotional and psychological well-being. If you like, you can do this movement for five to fifteen minutes.

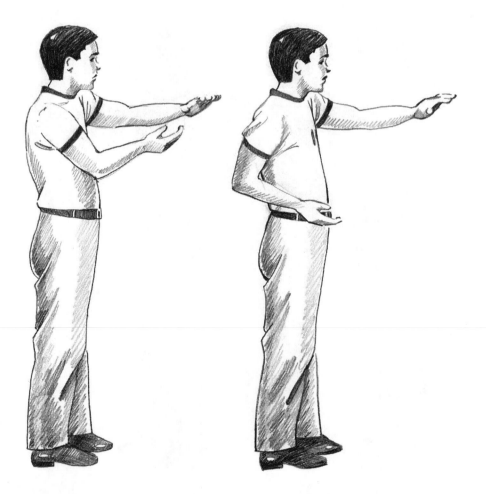

## EXERCISE 5:
## HOLDING THE CH'I AT THE DANTIEN

Widen your stance to about one and a half times the width of your shoulders. Imagine sitting on a shorter stool. This will help you tilt your pelvis forward slightly so that your spine remains straight. Place both hands, right over left, or left over right, on the Dantien, located three inches below the navel. Some people feel more comfortable with their right hand closest to the body. Some like the left hand closest to the body. Everyone is different. You can experiment to see which side feels more natural. After you have made this comparison,

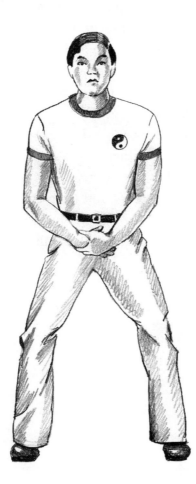

remember for future practice which one felt more comfortable.

Once your hands are situated, breathe naturally six times or for one or two minutes. If you feel good during this posture you can remain in it as long as you like. If you stand too long, though, you may experience shaking or aching in the legs, so don't force yourself. Hold this position for as long as it feels comfortable. The top of the head and the tailbone should be in a straight line. Make sure the breath is natural and effortless.

Keeping your palms overlapped in the same position, lift them two to four inches away from the Dantien. Rotate your palms around the Dantien six times in a clockwise direction. Repeat the rotation six times in a counter clockwise direction. Continue rotating six times in a clockwise direction, then six times in a counter clockwise direction until you have completed three repetitions in each direction. Be sure that the rotation is done slowly and gently.

The Dantien stores Ch'i. It expands and contracts as your internal energy is gathered and released. We must try to keep the tank full, but never stagnant. This form, practiced regularly, will move the Ch'i and keep the pathways through which the Ch'i flows clear. Ch'i is healing energy. If Ch'i is allowed to flow freely, good health results.

# PART 3

## THE MODERN WEST

# CHAPTER 13

# The Modern West

If there is one bridge that is fast emerging as the most fundamental link between the ancient East and the modern West, it is food. While the concept of food as therapy has long been disregarded by the modern West, it was one of the original eight sacred healing therapies of the ancient Chinese. Established some 6,000 years ago, food medicine is said to have been introduced by the great leader Shen Wung. Today, through the growing science of nutrition, the modern West is finally embracing the medicinal qualities of food. With this, the ancient Chinese teachings have come full circle to flower anew in the modern West. With more than 6,000 nutritional studies being conducted annually, we are at long last becoming aware of the profound impact that food plays in healing and disease.

Nutritional science first began to gain the respect of the modern West through evidence that linked dietary fats, most specifically cholesterol, with an increased risk in heart disease and high blood pressure. Since that time, nutritional science has more solidly established the therapeutic value of healthy foods in reversing a host of degenerative diseases. The latest information involves the discovery of previously unidentified medicinal food compounds called phytonutrients.

The public's desire for this knowledge is reflected in the immense amount of coverage the popular press gives these nutritional studies. Micro-nutrients, such as vitamins, minerals, trace minerals, proteins, fats, carbohydrates, amino acids, essential fatty acids,  and, most recently, phytonutrients, are among the list of those natural healing superstars we keep hearing about. Almost daily, new studies reveal a different food's ability to enhance health, healing, longevity, peak performance, and youthfulness. Pick up any magazine or newspaper and see the headlines: "Anti-aging Breakthrough," "Sleep Better With Natural Remedies," or "Ease Allergies Without Drugs." The modern West has, quite by surprise, made food its new super medicine. In this it has built a bridge from its scientific home base to the intuitive wisdom of the ancient East.

Today, the modern West is taking up where the first nutritionists left off so long ago, and at last there is an open flow of communication from both East and West. The modern West is no longer a one-dimensional mechanistic information base. It is at last demonstrating a willingness to consider more options. Because of this, many futurists project that alternative medicine, specifically nutrition, has the most profound potential for growth of any area in the new millennia. This isn't surprising when you consider how much we Westerners prize independence and self-control. These qualities are very much in keeping with the tenets of nutritional therapy, including responsibility for one's own health, illness prevention, the cultivation of peak performance, and longevity — with far fewer side-effects! In short, nutritional science holds the key to the future. What those of the ancient East knew in their hearts, the people of the modern West have discovered through their intellect. And, in the spirit of wholism, East and West will, by working together, usher health and natural healing into the new millenium.

# CHAPTER 14

# Basic Dietary Principles for Maximum Healing

## IT ALL BEGINS WITH DIGESTION

Creating vibrant health begins with good digestion, yet Americans spend two billion dollars each year on antacids. And while taking alkalizers may relieve the discomfort of heart burn, it does nothing to aid digestion. It is all well and good to eat healthy foods, but if your digestion is inadequate you will get little benefit from even the most nutritious diet. To take it a step further, I believe poor digestion is one of the the root causes of most degenerative illnesses.

What we think of as digestion can be more accurately described as the seven stages of food transformation. These stages, which accomplish the transformation of foods into compounds the body can use, include ingestion, digestion, absorption, transportation, respiration, metabolism, and excretion. The digestive breakdown process is both mechanical (chewing, muscular contraction, and peristalsis) and chemical (digestive enzymes breaking down the food into usable substances). The transformation of food is accomplished in the 25 to 30 foot long gastrointestinal tract, which extends from the mouth to the anus.

The process begins with ingestion in the mouth, where chewing increases the surface area of a bite-sized piece of food, thus creating more access for digestive enzymes to do their work. Several glands produce mylase and ptyalin, digestive enzymes designed to break down starches (or carbohydrates). It is interesting to note that carbohydrates are the first food group to begin to be digested, which suggests that the quick energy they provide helps fuel the long and laborious process we refer to simply as digestion.

From the mouth, the partially digested food travels through the esophagus to the stomach by the action of gravity and peristalsis, an involuntary wave-like muscular motion. In the stomach, food mixes with hydrochloric acid and pepsin which begins the process of breaking down fats and proteins.

A valve-like structure called the cardiac sphincter controls the entrance of food into the stomach and also prevents hydrochloric acid from splashing back up into the esophagus. When there is trouble in this area, it can often feel as though the pain is coming from the heart. Furthermore, indigestion of this type can initiate hiatal hernias and heart arrythmia.

From the stomach, food enters the small intestine, which is approximately 20 feet long and has three major sections. It is the work of the small intestine to finish digesting all three food groups. Although the liver, gallbladder, and pancreas are not part of the gastrointestinal tract, they each contribute to digestion by secreting substances into the small intestine that are essential to the process. The liver produces bile for fat emulsification, while the gallbladder stores bile from the liver and is also capable of secreting it into the small intestine as needed. The pancreas secretes a variety of enzymes that are essential for the digestion of fats, carbohydrates, and proteins. It is in the small intestine that nutrients are absorbed from the gastrointestinal tract into the blood and the lymph systems, which distribute them throughout the body.

From the small intestine, the non-digestible remnants, or ash, of the food we eat pass into the large intestine, or colon. Solid wastes are formed here, which contain food residue, bacteria, yeast, fungi, dead cells, cholesterol, and unabsorbed minerals. No digestion occurs here. This waste then collects in the rectum and passes from the body via the anal canal.

### STRESS AND PH

All of our mind-bodies move and change through time in sync with a number of cyclical rhythms triggered by light, temperatures, and certain internal phenomena. Among them are a 7-day biorhythmic cycle and a 28-day cycle. We also have a 24-hour metabolic cycle, during which certain hours are favored for particular body functions. For instance, digestion is best accomplished by the body between the hours of 7 a.m. and 3 p.m., while tissue building takes place between 3 p.m. and 11 p.m. The third cycle, which occurs between the hours of 11 p.m. and 7 a.m., is when the body naturally cleanses cellular wastes.

One of the most important cycles in terms of health is the pH (potential Hydrogen) cycle, which measures the acid-alkaline chemical balance in the body. While it is normal for the body's pH to fluctuate as part of a daily pH cycle, our acid-alkaline balance must remain within a narrow range in order to sustain life. Within this narrow range, there is an optimum balance point which indicates a healthy state. pH is measured in all the body fluids, with blood pH being the principle guiding indicator. Blood pH should range from between

7.2–7.4. If yours is below 7.2, you are far too acid and most likely very ill, and if it is above 7.4 you are far too alkaline and also likely to be very ill. A balanced pH indicates a healing state, while excesses in either extreme indicate an environment ripe for disease.

The easiest vehicle for monitoring pH is urine. The scale for urine pH is different from that of blood, but it corresponds with blood's. Urine pH ranges from 5.0–7.0, with the healthy balance point between 6.4–6.8. Thus, a urinary pH of 6.4–6.8 tells you that your blood pH is exactly balanced between 7.3 and 7.4. Urinary pH that is consistently well below 6.4 indicates a very acidic, fiery condition in the body. This reflects a hyper-stress environment that predisposes a person toward illnesses such as rheumatoid arthritis, diabetes, lupus, fibromyalgia, and a variety of cancers. On the other hand, a urinary pH consistently well above 6.8 indicates an hyper-alkaline environment that usually reflects a broken down, deficient condition caused by extreme stress over a long period of time. This predisposes a person to melancholia, diarrhea, heart disease, indigestion, and immune deficiency.

Most of us these days suffer from overly acidic conditions. Stress causes the body to produce stress hormones and other acids which contribute to this. Clearly, controlling stress is key to bringing an acidic pH into balance. From a more mechanical perspective, eating at least two large servings of chlorophyll-rich, green, leafy vegetables each day will help a hyper-acid pH. On the other hand, over-indulging in processed, high-starch, dead carbohydrates and fatty proteins tends to create acidic conditions. (For information on testing urine pH and ways to neutralize pH and bring it into a state of balance, please see the notes at the end of the chapter.)

Since stress plays such large role in creating disease and blocking health, I would like to drive the point home to you by outlining what I believe to be the dynamics of the stress response. So many of us use the words stress and stressed-out frequently, but few of us know what it actually means.

## FIGHT OR FLIGHT STRESS RESPONSE
### *(General Adaptation Syndrome)*

Fight or flight, or the stress response, evolved to help ancient human beings adapt to the world they lived in. Primitive cave dwellers, who encountered a number of life and death situations, needed to be able to respond fast and powerfully to sudden events. The stress response gave them the energy they needed to accomplish feats they would have been unable to accomplish under normal circumstances.

Although we moderns don't have to outsmart a sabre-toothed tiger or run from a mastodon, we are equipped with the same response system that our primitive ancestors had. Interestingly, it doesn't matter what the stressful situation actually is that shifts us into the fight or flight mode. What matters is how we *perceive* or *interpret* the situation. Whatever we see as threatening, what we become anxious about, what makes us angry or impatient, all serve to patch us through to the circuits that turn on the stress response. Instantaneously, such perceptions activate chemical messages that travel from the brain's hypothalamus, pineal gland, amygdala, and the sensory cortex — throughout the body. These chemical messages communicate an entirely different set of instructions than the ones used for healthy, normal living (homeostasis). In this stress condition, the body's priority is to manufacture as much energy as it can as fast as it can. All other functions not crucial to producing immediate energy in response to the perceived emergency are suspended.

The second, the hypothalamus (our stress sensor) perceives the initial stress, the pituitary gland activates the adrenal glands to produce a number of stress hormones that begin the first of three stages of redirecting physiological activities.

In the first (acute) stage of alarm reaction, the adrenal hormones send the message to the body to increase the heart rate to prepare the body machine for increased inertia. Next, the peripheral blood vessels in the hands, feet, and skin are constricted so that the internal vital organs can receive more blood. Then, the spleen contracts and blood clotting increases to offset any potential for excessive bleeding. The liver's glycogen stores are released so as to increase the energy supply. Sweat production is then increased to lower the rising body temperature. Breathing steps up, and the respiratory passageways expand to facilitate oxygen intake which in turn allows the body to eliminate the excess carbon dioxide from catabolism (tissue breakdown for energy). Finally, saliva and enzyme releases are decreased as digestion is not necessary.

Then, if stress persists, the second resistance response (chronic stress) stage engages. Through the colinergic response, large stores of hydrochloric acid are released which are designed to burn food quickly so the body can fight, or flee, more efficiently. This causes blood pH to become very acidic which is conducive to the energy burning function that becomes the body's top priority during the stress response.

Having burned through its food sources, the body then begins to withdraw protein from the thymus and lymph glands to break *it* down for use as immediate energy. Quite a bit of calcium is lost through this process, since almost 50% of the body's calcium is bonded with proteins, which, remember, act as the body's Public Works Department, constantly fixing and repairing the body. During the stress response, all normal repair and maintenance work is suspended, as the body diverts all proteins for use as energy. This withdrawal of protein from these critical glands is a powerfully destructive process.

Additionally, excess sugars store in the liver as starch or glycogen, ready to be instantly reconverted to energy on demand.

As part of this process, blood pressure rises to facilitate the flow of energy to vital organs. Because the normal work of proteins is halted, the body withdraws minerals from the bones to use for repair work. More calcium, so crucial to strong bones, is lost in this way, as are other minerals, including magnesium, so essential for calming nerves. Again, the body is almost cannibalizing itself to mobilize all the energy it can to respond to the stress situation. Fat is also called upon to be used as quick energy and sodium is retained in order to help the body hold on to its water reserves to prevent dehydration.

As I have said, the fight or flight response was designed to be used in emergency situations lasting very short periods of time. It is essential that it be turned off as soon as possible to allow the body to return to its normal health-maintaining activities. The stress response wasn't meant to go on for long periods of time. Thus, when the stress response becomes chronic, we end up depleting all the excess reserves in our organs. We can no longer pull protein from exhausted glands because there is none left, nor take calcium from broken-down bone tissue.

In this stage, the body has shifted to another strategy to get the immediate energy it needs. This is accomplished by diverting every bit of food for use as immediate energy. Normally, a portion of food is used immediately, while the rest goes into a number of building and storing processes. Among these are the maintenance of the immune system; routine repair work; and the routine storage of energy for future use. During this stage of the stress response, none of these normal and important activities can take place because the body, having depleted all its reserves, has nowhere to turn for energy except the food that it eats. Once Stage Two becomes chronic, the body becomes completely exhausted and passes into a Stage Three state of acute stress response. At this point, the mind–body is extremely depleted and deficient. This is a state of extreme exhaustion that can sometimes lead to death.

## STRESS DIGESTION

As I've emphasized, stress has a powerfully damaging effect on the mind–body, which includes digestion. When experts talk about digestion. or writers describe it in text-books, they refer to digestion in an ideal person who lives a peaceful life and has a calm mind–body. Unfortunately, this applies to few modern Americans. Our bodies were designed to live in a calm, sympathetic-dominant state of being 90% of the time, with the capacity to shift into the fight or flight stress response mode approximately 10% of the time, as needed. Unfortunately, today, it is just the opposite, with the vast major-ity of us spending a good 90% of our time in a stressed, fight or flight mode, and 10% of our time feeling relaxed and easy.

Because of this, I hold that there are two kinds of diges-tion. One is the healthy digestion of a mostly stress-free person, and the other is the digestion of the acutely stressed, which I refer to as Stress Digestion. Eating a wonderful diet will do little for you if you are in a acute state of stress.

Chronic Stage Two stress causes the body to over-pro-duce hydrochloric acid to burn through food very quickly in order to sustain the emergency stress mode. The chronic over-production of hydrochloric acid, however, depletes these digestive juices, leaving inadequate stores for later use. Yet, without hydrochloric acid we cannot begin to digest proteins, fats, calciums, and a number of other substances, which impairs digestion immeasurably. Consequently, partially digested proteins end up putrefying in the large intestines, while partially digested carbohydrates ferment. In theory, foods such as broccoli have the potential to be powerfully medicinal, but any food that stays in the body longer than the normal transit period of 28–36 hours becomes a pathogen. Impaired digestion leads the way to numerous degenerative diseases that have many names with which we are all too familiar. But this is only the half of it. Just as chronic stress suppresses the production of the digestive aid hydrochloric acid, it also produces enormous neuroendocrine imbalances throughout the body which impact the digestive process by affecting the blood pressure as well as the heart, liver, gall bladder, intestines, and pancreas.

As I've said, fight or flight is geared toward supplying the mind–body with extra energy. It accomplishes much of this through the combined action of the adrenal hormones which redirect the action of most of the body's systems from all functions not essential to survival. In doing so, they also stimulate cardiac function, increasing the rate and force of the heart's contractions, raise blood pressure, and dilate blood vessels. In addition, they activate enzymes that promote glucose formation in the liver, while inhibiting the pancreatic production of insulin. Decreased insulin prevents glucose from being used by the tissue and increases its availability to the central nervous system. The adrenal hormones also mobilize fats for use in the fight, and inhibit the breakdown of cholesterol.

Chronic adrenaline release raises blood glucose levels, increasing the risk of adult onset diabetes and hypoglycemia. It also speeds respiratory and metabolic rates, which increases the risk of thyroid and parathyroid problems. Additionally, chronic adrenaline release constricts the blood vessels in the intestine further, hampering protein digestion and assimilation, while dilating blood vessels in the muscles, which raises the risk of musculo-skeleton debilitation. The depletion of adrenaline from chronic stress also destroys adrenaline's ability to function as an anti-inflammatory crucial to the neutralization of allergic and inflammatory reactions.

Through the combined working of all aspects of this stress response, a wide array of enzymes and hormones responsible for regulating normal processes are suppressed, including sex hormone production, digestive enzyme production, and the production and circulation of lymphocytes, white blood cells, and other components of the immune system. Additionally, stress adversely affects the cardiovascular system, bone density, wound repair, brain function, and genetic integrity.

### A PATIENT'S STORY

One of my patients, I will call him William, came to me when he was in his early 30's. He was 6'1" and had weighed 138 pounds his entire adult life. No matter what he tried, everything from protein powders to high-fat, high carbohydrate foods, he couldn't gain any weight. A while after I met William, he bought his first house and then almost immediately he lost his job. Suddenly, he was thrown into an acute state of stress; after having a secure source of money, he had no income for the first time in his life. He was terribly worried that he wouldn't be able to make his house payments.

In a very short time, William shot up to 220 pounds. This marked weight gain was the result of a change in the activity of his thyroid. Normally responsible for controlling fatty metabolism, William's thyroid had previously been overactive. After the onset of his stress, however, his routine thyroid activity was diverted from its normal metabolic functioning to support the needs of the stress response. Thus, his thyroid became underactive as a calorie burning mechanism and he gained nearly 80 pounds.

## MORE ON STRESS DIGESTION

The preceding illustrations reflect just a smattering of the functions that become disrupted and neglected during the fight or flight response. What is essential to understand is that this response is designed to last short periods of time to allow the body to respond to an acute, emergency situation. It was and is essential to wellness that this potentially destructive mode be turned off as soon as possible. Clearly, stress is not just something that makes us a little tired. It is a very real, potentially destructive force. Unfortunately, modern life and our often unconscious decision to go fast, get more, and generally "keep up with the Joneses" has caused many of us to live in a near-constant state of fight or flight. It is up to each one of us to become more committed to peace of mind and body in our lives. In order to be available to the medicinal qualities of food, we need to shift out of stress digestion into a normal, healthy, stress-free digestion capable of delivering the essential nutrients on which our minds and bodies depend.

## BIO-INDIVIDUALITY: NO DIET IS RIGHT FOR EVERYONE ALL THE TIME

It is important to understand that because we each have specific and unique nutritional needs, no single diet is right for everyone. Additionally, each person is subject to constantly changing conditions, and what might be good for you during one period might not be so good for you during another.

The earlier chapters on the Five Constitutional Types introduced you to the concept of individual Constitutional Types as used by various cultures including the ancient Chinese, Indian, Arabic, and classical Greek. These systems, used to differentiate among people's unique constitutions, helped individuals and healers to better understand the energetic nature of a person and his or her corresponding tendencies, strengths, and weaknesses. Knowing if we are high strung and tend toward excitability, or whether we are more likely to withdraw, feel cold, and have little appetite helps to tailor our diets to the foods that are best for our individual constitutions.

This bio-individuality accounts for the fact that so many widely differing, often contrary, diet systems are popular today; some are good for some people and some are good for others. Popular diets that emphasize protein, others that stress carbohydrates, and others still that recommend only raw foods, are all valid and valuable for some Types and not for others. I feel that it is essential, then, that each person find a way to tailor the following basic dietary guidelines to their particular constitutions and intolerances (allergic reactions). I use both the Five Constitutional Types that are presented in earlier chapters, as well as AK (Applied Kinesiology) testing — a system that reads the body's subtle electrical muscular responses to determine if a particular food is tolerable for a person at a particular time. There are a number of other means, both esoteric and mechanical, to determine your individual nutritional approach and what foods are best for you, including Vega testing, food rotation, Elisa testing and cytotoxic or scratch testing.

If you are working with the Five Constitutional Types, you may want to modify the basic diet by using more foods from the Food Flavor group that corresponds with your Type. For example, if you are a Fire Type in a high-energy mode you will want to use more bitter vegetables (good for reducing inflammatory conditions) rather than a full range of vegetables. If, on the other hand, you are a Water Type in an exhausted state, you may need to increase your intake of protein foods. There is always room to adjust the basic dietary guidelines to adapt better to the changing needs in your life.

The following section presents several aspects of the basic dietary guidelines that I believe to be the fundamental starting point for a healthy diet. These guidelines are intended for use when you're feeling fine. When and if you are ill or experiencing an acute health crisis, I would recommend a more strictly medicinal diet under a doctor's care. I will explain further as we go on.

## THE BASIC PROGRAM

To begin with, I categorize all foods into one of three major groups. The first group, *toxic foods*, includes all processed sugary and snack junk foods, and also the highly carcinogenic cured deli meats and bacon. The toxic food group also includes all intolerable, allergenic foods. It is important to realize that each of us has different food intolerances and allergies unique to us. Often we think we don't have any allergies if we don't have typical allergic reactions, but food intolerances and allergies can have less obvious, though equally debilitating, effects. Food intolerances can be the cause of headaches, backaches, indigestion and a wide array of other health problems.

The second group, *neutral foods*, are those foods which are not directly disease-producing, but which have no healing potential, such as white pasta and white rice. The third group, *medicinal foods*, includes a wide range of fruits and vegetables, whole grains, legumes, and certain lean protein sources that are not allergenic to you.

As a general guideline, I recommend that people strive to consume a ratio of at least 70% medicinal foods, and no more than 15% each of the neutral and toxic groups. I call this my 85% rule, which suggests that you strive to eat wholesome (neutral or medicinal) foods 85% of the time.

I also break foods down into three categories in terms of individual digestion. The first group I call tolerance foods, which are those foods that we can eat on a daily basis and digest well. The second category are swing foods — those foods that a person is able to digest only on an occasional basis. (Eating too much of a swing food often pushes it into the intolerance category, while abstaining from it for a period may allow you to regain your tolerance.) Finally, intolerance foods are those which act as allergens to a person. No matter how little you eat of an intolerance food, you cannot digest it. About 65% of the average person's diet is comprised of tolerance foods, about 25% swing foods, and about 10% are intolerance foods.

Having divided foods into these three categories, I then make my dietary recommendations according to food groups. I recommend that 65% of your daily caloric intake be comprised of whole, unrefined grains and grain products (brown rice, rye, oats, millet, quinoa), vegetables, and fruits. Twenty to 25% of the diet should be from fats, the majority of which should be mono and polyunsaturated. Finally, 12-15% should be comprised of low-fat animal and vegetable proteins. (It is important to keep in mind that these percentages are general guidelines; each person should be screened to determine his or her individual needs using one of the aforementioned techniques.) I also recommend that fruits be eaten more frequently when they are in season — between May and November in temperate climates.

Food preparation, too, should be adjusted to be in balance with the seasons so that cold, raw foods are served more in the late spring and summer, while warm, cooked foods are preferred in the fall and winter. Cooking methods and the use of raw versus cooked foods can also be determined by the Constitutional Type of the person and his or her needs at a particular time. (For this information, please see earlier chapters.) In general, however, I recommend cooked foods over raw, as proper cooking destroys pathogens while increasing many nutrient yields and decreasing phlegm production in the body. Additionally, cooking methods — baking, broiling, sautéing, poaching, braising and boiling — should be varied to produce a varied abundance of nutrients.

## CLEANING OUT THE KITCHEN CABINETS

Because the following items tend to fall into the toxic and intolerant food category, I recommend avoiding them whenever possible:

— All sugars: sucrose, dextrose, glucose, maltose, corn sweeteners, turbinado sugar, raisin syrup, honey, maple syrup, molasses, and anything made from them.

— Any and all fried foods; white flour products and other processed carbohydrates including white rice, buns, rolls, sweet rolls, doughnuts, pizza, crackers, chewing gum (sugar-free or otherwise), soft drinks, (sugar-free or otherwise), cake, cookies, icecream, white flour pasta, sweetened juices, condiments such as mayonnaise, ketchup, relish, jellies, jams, gravies, excessively fatty foods such as sour cream, cream soups, chowders, alcohol, and caffeinated drinks of any kind.

Additionally, I generally recommend that wheat, corn, and dairy be reduced because of their high concentration of allergens. Similarly, yeasted breads and baked goods should be replaced with yeast-free, sour dough products; vinegars should be replaced with molkosan (a liquid whey), or sulfite-free lemon and lime juices. Additionally, all fermented soy-type sauces should be replaced with Bragg's Amino Liquid, which is very much similar in taste and function to soy sauce, and peanuts and peanut butters should be replaced with almonds and almond butters. (Peanuts contain the potentially toxic aflatoxin mold, while almonds are aflatoxin-free.) I believe that the above-mentioned fermented foods increase the risk of escalating the populations of immuno-suppressive yeast in the body.

## FOOD COMBINING

Over the years, there have been many studies substantiating the value of eating certain food groups *with* certain food groups, and not with others. Most notable is the work of Dr. Herbert M. Shelton, who compiled extensive research on the topic from 1928 to 1981. Dr. Shelton's research was first noted in 1924 in the *Journal of American Medicine* by Dr. Philip Norman, who cited the effectiveness of proper food combining. My professional experience has led me to concur with this theory. I continually see the remarkable healing power of proper food combining, especially for those patients whose problems are traceable to digestive or metabolic difficulties.

Properly combined foods digest efficiently, whereas improperly combined foods may upset healthy digestion and nutrient assimilation. This is because different enzymes are required to break down various foods, and they can interfere with each other, causing cause nitrogen, methane, and hydrogen gases to ferment in the intestines. The following Food Combining chart encapsulates the fundamentals of proper food combining.

**PROTEINS**
**(1 per meal)**
beans, dairy, eggs,
fish, nuts, legumes,
meat, poultry, soy

**YES**

**Low Starch**
**VEGETABLES**
celery, garlic, okra, onions,
peppers, summer squash,
asparagus, broccoli,
leafy greens

**NO**

**YES**

**High Starch VEGETABLES**
beets, carrots, corn, parsnips, peas, potatoes, pumpkin, yams

**High Starch GRAINS**
breads, cereals, crackers, pastas, rice

| Acid **FRUITS** | Sub Acid **FRUITS** | Sweet **FRUITS** |
|---|---|---|
| citrus, pineapple, kiwi, strawberry, tomato | apple, apricot, berries, cherries, grapes, melons, nectarine, pear, oranges, peach, papaya, plum | bananas, currants, dates, figs, raisins |

**All fruits taken alone and combined only with their groupings**

## RULES

**1.** Only 1 protein per meal
**2.** Do not combine proteins with starches
**3.** Do not combine fruits with any other foods or any other fruit group
**4.** Proteins combine well with low starch vegetables
**5.** Low starch vegetables combine well with starch vegetables
★ Chew all food well
★ Take beverages before or two hours after meals — never during

## WHAT YOU SEE MAY NOT BE
## WHAT YOU GET

Although it is beyond the scope of this book to delve deeply into the issue of food purity, I would feel negligent if I failed to touch upon it.

As I've already discussed, many of us in the West don't believe something unless we can see it, measure it, or test it. Consequently, we think that if we can't see something, it can't hurt us. Sadly, there are many compounds in foods that we can't see, or taste, that have unhealthy effects on us. The truth is that if our goal is a healthy, whole state of being, we not only need to make choices concerning the foods we eat, but we also need to consider the quality of the foods themselves. If we know what farmers, producers, and manufacturers are doing to our food, we can make healthier choices at the market-place, thus registering our preferences and requirements with every dollar we spend. Should we feel so inclined, we can also be more vocal and active in the struggle to reclaim purer growing conditions for our food supply, and fight any addi-tional legislation that seeks to lower the standards that are meant to safeguard the quality of our foods.

### A BIT OF HISTORY

Until the mid-1940's, American farmers used natural means to return vital nutrients to the soil, a practice which ensured nutritious food. After the second World War, howev-er, things changed. Surplus chemicals used in the war, including nitrates and phosphates, found a use as low-cost, high-yield chemical fertilizers. By the early 1960's, the American farm industry had totally converted to the synthet-ic fertilizers we have today, depleting crops of vital nutrients.

Taking up where the farmer leaves off, manufacturers dry, salt, pickle, sugar, ferment, smoke, freeze, can, preserve, artificially supplement, and irradiate our foods. More damaging than these processes, however, are the arsenal of chemicals added to our foods to make them more appealing, including dyes, bleaches, emulsifiers, antioxidants, preservatives, flavor enhancers, buffers, sprays, acidifiers, alkalizers, deodorants, gases, drying agents, fortifiers, hydrolizers, anti-foaming agents, caking agents and hydrogenators.

Unbelievably, this is not the end of the story. The most damaging practices of all involve pesticides and fungicides. Among the most dangerous are those with chlorinated hydrocarbon chains, including DDT, endrin, aldrin and toxaphene. These chemicals don't break down, but rather continually re-cycle through food chains... and our bodies. Although DDT was banned by Congress in 1972, it continues to show up in dangerously high levels in certain seafoods. Many pesticides still in use today are sprayed regularly on virtually every fruit and vegetable you see at the market place. Independent studies consistently find a horrifying number of chemical residues in these foods. (To counteract some of these toxins, I recommend spritzing produce with two solutions. First use a mixture of 1 teaspoon cider vinegar in 10 ounces of water followed a mixture of 1 teaspoon of baking soda in 10 ounces of water. Use a final water rinse. There are also rinses available commercially at most natural foods stores.)

Ideally, the government should assure the safety of our food supply, but the issue becomes tainted by confused priorities and special interests. Not only that, but long-term human safety is unknown as are safe exposure levels. Yet it is the job of the Environmental Protection Agency (EPA) to determine the "tolerance levels" that are allowed for pesticide residues in foods, and the Food and Drug Administration, along with the Department of Agriculture, are responsible for enforcing these levels. The problem is that many scientists and researchers do not agree on what constitutes safe levels of these potentially dangerous toxins.

In 1993, The National Academy of Sciences (NAS) found that the legal tolerance levels of exposure to pesticides for particular foods is no guarantee of safety for children. A late 1980s report by The Natural Resources Defense Council (NRDC) concluded that nearly three million American children are exposed to higher levels of neurotoxic pesticides than the EPA considers acceptable. The NRDC concluded that 5,500 to 6,200 preschoolers may eventually develop cancer as a result of childhood exposure to pesticides. Furthermore, tolerance levels are set with adults in mind, and children's bodies have consistently demonstrated dramatically different tolerances and reaction responses. Despite the fact that the NAS found the entire EPA regulatory system lacking and inadequate, none of their recommendations have been adopted by the EPA, nor has Congress forced the EPA to do so.

Today, new processes are being developed and introduced that take the denaturalization of foods even further. Bovine Growth Hormone is now fed to dairy cows to make milk production higher. Frequently, this causes the animals to develop infected mammary glands requiring antibiotics that are then passed on to the consumer. Genetic alterations are also in the works, so that a tomato could possibly have animal genes in its flesh. Tragically, the law does not require the labeling of these products, so the only way you can be sure that the dairy you are getting is free of synthetic hormones, or the tomato is purely vegetarian, is to buy organic products.

Sadly, the most current fight involves just that — organic foods. The latest attack on those trying to ensure a clean and safe food supply involves the attempt to change the practices that qualify a food as organically grown. The most insidious of these changes would allow toxic sludges, the by-products of sewage treatment plants, to be used as fertilizers on so-called organic foods.

And it doesn't end with food. America's drinking water is almost exclusively fluoridated. Although we are continually reassured by science that fluoridation in no way jeopardizes our well being, there is mounting evidence to the contrary. The largest American study, involving more than 39,000 school children, concluded that fluoridation does not, in fact, reduce tooth decay in permanent teeth. Similar studies have taken place in New Zealand and Canada with similar results. Despite this, fluoride continues to appear in a number of products aside from our water supply, and consequently all of our drinks, and cooked foods.

Fluoride has been readily documented as a toxic compound which many world-wide studies have linked to osteoporosis, arthritis, skeletal flourosis, collagen breakdown, genetic birth defects, and cancer. One such study by Williams and Williams,★ published in 1984, stated unequivocally that fluoride was more poisonous than lead, and just slightly less toxic than arsenic. Best-selling author Harvey Diamond reports in his book *Fit for Life II*, "According to Dr. Dean Burke, former chief biochemist at the National Cancer Institute, more than 50,000 Americans a year are dying of cancer caused by fluoridated drinking water." Dr. Burke made these statements on June 18, 1985 at an EPA environmental hearing.

Clearly, it is important to be aware of the adulteration of our food and water supply, so that we can make the best choices about what we eat and feed our families and friends. Organically grown foods are now much more widely available in conventional supermarkets, and natural food stores everywhere. There is also a ground swell of farmer's markets in nearly every town and city that offer foods grown with fewer dangerous compounds.

Just as we seek balance in all things, we need to balance our response to this problem. I suggest doing your best to get the purest foods you can, while learning about the issues.

NOTE: To test your urinary pH, I recommend using the .067 pHydrion paper strips, that measure urine pH from 5.5–8.0. They are available in health food stores and some pharmacies, and are made by Micro Essential Laboratory, Inc., in Brooklyn, N.Y. 11210. Test your first urine of the day by letting it run across a several inch strip of the pHydrion paper, then immediately compare the color to the chart on the container.

To regulate an overly acid pH you can try the following, depending on your bio-individuality and the state of your constitution:
Cold baths and showers
Deep breathing
Yoga exercise
Ta'i Ch'i
Fresh vegetable juice
Raw salads
Lemon juice and water
Herb teas, especially alfalfa
Chlorophyll capsules: (2) twice a day
Epsom salt baths
Aerobic exercise

To regulate an overly alkaline pH you can try the following, depending on your bio-individuality and the state of your constitution:

Papain-bromalain enzymes

Multi-digestive enzymes

Raw acid foods, including pineapple, papaya, and grapefruit

Herbal teas, especially spearmint

Brisk walks

Hot baths and showers

# CHAPTER 15

# Fighting Cancer and Heart Disease with Food:

## *The Magnificent Seven Phytonutrients and the Top 25 Foods*

### THE HEALING POWER OF FOODS

The vitamins and minerals in our foods have long been known to be capable of preventing a variety of diseases. Today, the most exciting new research substantiating the powerful healing properties of food involves a new category of previously unidentified medicinal compounds in fruits and vegetables called phytonutrients. These compounds, used by plants to protect themselves against various environmental stresses, have been found to have drug-like powers to both reverse disease and prevent it. To date, seven families of phytonutrients, each of which contain hundreds of different compounds, have been identified. All fruits and vegetables each contain a variety of phytonutrients, which act synergistically to most beneficially deliver the therapeutic compounds they contain. In other words, whole foods are engineered by Nature to contain all the co-compounds necessary for the body to best utilize a particular food's medicinal formulas.

## THE ANTIOXIDANT PROPERTIES OF PHYTONUTRIENTS

Among the phytonutrient's most valuable properties is its ability to act as an antioxidant (those substances that counteract free radical damage). In simple terms, free-radicals are molecules that are missing an electron due to pollution, stress, or a variety of other natural and unnatural conditions. Because free radicals need an electron, they attack healthy cells and steal theirs, thus damaging the healthy cells. To make matters worse, this theft turns the newly-attacked cells into electron-lacking, free radicals also, creating a chain reaction that can cause cancer, heart disease, and other untold damage. In their quest to quench their thirst for an electron, free radicals attack all cells, including those in our genes.

Genes, made of DNA, are responsible for instructing our cells how to behave; when DNA is strong and healthy, we are strong and healthy. However, DNA is comprised of long strands of molecules which are easily damaged. Some of that damage occurs as a result of natural processes, but the majority of it is caused by free radicals which mutate, or alter, DNA's original, perfect, code. Eventually, if there is enough mutation, the instructions and information encoded within the DNA become so distorted that it can no longer send healthy operating instructions to our cells, which results in disease. Experts concur that upwards of 90% of all cancers result from mutated DNA, as well as heart disease and virtually all other degenerative diseases.

Because of this, antioxidant-rich, free-radical-fighting phytonutrients are now considered to be on the cutting edge of disease prevention and reversal!

# THE MAGNIFICENT SEVEN PHYTONUTRIENTS

## Carotenoids

Carotenoids, the first of our phytonutrient families, all share the red and yellow pigments that we see in carrots, tomatoes, and other fruits and vegetables. To date, more than 600 different carotenoids have been identified. Among them are *lutein, zeaxanthan, alpha,* and *gamma,* as well as the family's most prized members, *lycopene* and *beta carotene.*

*Lycopene,* most abundantly found in cooked tomatoes, is a powerful antioxidant. A Harvard study of 48,000 men found that those who ate 10 half-cup servings of cooked tomatoes cut their risk of prostate cancer by 48%. Researchers at Dana Farber Cancer Institute and Harvard Medical School, evaluating the prostate tissue of 25 men, also determined that tomato consumption was linked with a lowered incidence of prostate cancer.[*] Lycopene has also been implicated in reductions in the risk of colon, rectal, and stomach cancers. It is important to note that cooking tomatoes greatly increases the availability of lycopene. *Beta-carotene,* most commonly found in apricots, carrots, cantaloupe, yams, sweet potatoes, and winter squash, has been found to lower the risk of a variety of cancers. Recent studies have found that subjects who had the highest amounts of beta carotene in their diet had a significantly lower risk of death from cancer.

Other studies have confirmed that various carotenoids in green leafy vegetables, such as kale, spinach, and broccoli, significantly lower the risk of macular degeneration — the leading cause of eye disease in people over 50. The most potent sources of carotenoids are tomatoes, carrots, broccoli,

---

[*] Selene Yeager and the editors of PREVENTION MAGAZINE, *New Foods For Healing: Capture the Powerful Cures of More than 100 Common Foods.* Rodale Press, Inc. Emmaus, PA, 1998

and greens. It is important to note that the absorption of caratenoids is enhanced by eating some fatty acids with them, such as olive oil.

### Flavinoids

Flavinoids, our second family of phytonutrients, include *quercetin, anthocyanins, rutin,* and *hesperdin.* Flavinoids are found most abundantly in apples, berries, apricots, onions, purple grapes, endive, kale, and red wine. Along with flavinoid's antioxidant properties, they are also powerful heart protectors that help thin the blood, protecting against the formation of blood clots.

Recent laboratory studies have established that the flavinoids in red wine could, in some cases, prevent up to 100% of LDL (bad) blood cholesterol from oxidizing, and thus from clotting. Among other studies, flavinoids have been found to halt the progression of colon tumors in animals, lower the risk of stomach cancers, and reduce brain dysfunction and memory loss.

### Monoterpenes

Monoterpenes, our third family of phytonutrients, include such compounds are *limonene,* found most abundantly in citrus oils and peels. *Perillyl alcohol* is another monoterpene that has garnered attention in recent years.

Monterpenes appear to have a special ability to fight the formation of cancerous tumors. Recent university medical studies have established that laboratory animals given a limited diet of *limonene* showed a significant reduction in cancerous tumors. Elsewhere, researchers have established that limonene consistently encouraged cancer cells to self-destruct. Other studies have consistently shown limonene to increase the activity of proteins that eliminate estradiol — a hormone linked to breast cancer.

*Perillyl alcohol,* another monoterpene, has consistently demonstrated the ability to block cancers of the breast, lungs, stomach, liver, pancreas and skin.

### Polyphenolic Compounds

This group of phytonutrients includes *catechins, curcurmin* and *ellagic acid*. Polyphenols are found most abundantly in green and black teas, all berries, olive oil, most vegetables, whole grains, and turmeric. Polyphenols have demonstrated profound anti-cancer effects; researchers have established that ellagic acid reduces free radicals and detoxifies carcinogens. Meanwhile, other scientists are finding that the ellagic acid in olive oil provided powerful protection against free-radicals, protecting both the arteries and breasts, lowering the risk of female breast cancers by as much as 25%!

### Indoles and Isothiocyanates

Our fifth group of phytonutrients include *Indole 3 Carbinol* (I3C's) and *sulforaphane*. They are most abundantly found in broccoli, brussels sprouts, cabbage, cauliflower, and mustard greens.

Scientists have discovered I3C's to work as agents that sweep up the body's excess harmful estrogens before they can contribute to cancer cell development, while increasing levels of healthy faux-estrogens. A variety of population studies have shown I3C's to be useful as protective agents against colon, breast, prostate, and cervical cancers.

Many oncology researchers are concluding that sulforaphan triggers the release of enzymes that rid the body of toxins, reducing the risk of free radical damage and cancer.

## Allylic Sulfides

Our sixth group of phytonutrients are most abundantly found in garlic and onions. Among them are the compounds *diallyl disulfide* (DADS), and *diallyl trisulfide.*

In one recent study, male subjects with elevated cholesterol were given a garlic extract rich in allylic sulfides. Many of the patients had as much as a 60% decrease in their platelet counts. Many similar studies are continually finding these compounds to be effective blood thinners, thus reducing the risk of heart disease.

Substances in garlic have been shown to slow the development of prostate cancer cells and studies also suggest that certain of its active ingredients may also lower cholesterol, bring down high blood pressure, boost the immune system, and block carcinogens in foods eaten with garlic.★

## Isoflavones

The most well-known of our last group of phytonutrients are isoflavones, which contain the currently popular *genistein* and *daidzein* which are found abundantly in soybeans and their products, as well as chick peas, kidney beans, and lentils.

Among the most powerful actions of isoflavones is their ability to act as regulators of hormones. Currently, many American women are using soy products to help mitigate the unpleasant effects of menopause and pre-menopause. Isoflavones help prevent harmful estrogens from attaching to cell receptors by attaching to the receptors themselves, thus blocking the action of the harmful estrogens such as cancer causing 16 Alpha Hydroxy Esterone. In study after study we are seeing the documented evidence that isoflavones are clearly reducing the risk of breast cancers. Studies have shown that women had significantly fewer hot flashes after three months of eating an ounce and a half of soy flour daily. Japanese women, who traditionally eat much soy, have one of the lowest incidences of breast cancer in the world. Several studies have documented this.

Isoflavones are also particularly good at lowering LDL cholesterol, and, once again, soy is an excellent source from which to get this substance, and is most beneficial if substituted for animal protein in the diet.

Clearly, foods have wondrous healing properties that science is just beginning to uncover. Vegetables and fruits, in particular, are powerful healers. Make use of them and help yourself to Nature's offerings. How many servings have you had today?

---

* NOTE: Some of the above research specifics were culled from PREVENTION's *New Foods For Healing*

## MY TOP 25
## PHYTONUTRIENT-RICH
## SUPER-FOODS

| Food | Phytonutrient |
|------|---------------|
| Tomatoes | Carotenoids |
| Apricots | Carotenoids; Flavinoids |
| Chicory | Carotenoids |
| Brussels Sprouts | Indoles/ Isothiocyanates |
| Cabbage | Indoles/ Isothiocyanates |
| Broccoli | Carotenoids; Indoles/ Isothiocyanates |
| Sweet potatoes/ yams: | Carotenoids |
| Blueberries | Flavinoids; Polyphenols |
| Purple grapes | Flavinoids; Polyphenols |
| Red Wine | Flavinoids; Polyphenols |
| Olive Oil *(cold, first pressed, extra virgin)* | Polyphenols |

| Food | Phytonutrient |
| --- | --- |
| Granny Smith Apples | Flavinoids |
| Onions | Allylic Sulfides |
| Garlic | Allylic Sulfides |
| Lemons | Monoterpenes |
| Oranges | Monoterpenes; Flavinoids |
| Cherries | Monoterpenes |
| Tumeric | Polyphenols |
| Black pepper | Polyphenols |
| Tofu | Isoflavinoids |
| Black beans | Isoflavinoids |
| Oatmeal | Tocotrienols |
| Green tea | Polyphenols |
| Salmon | EFAs |
| Strawberries | Polyphenols |
| Celery | |

# CHAPTER 16

# Supplementing
# the Fight Against Disease

*Vitamins, Minerals and Other*
*Natural Medicines*

I recently read that Americans take 2.5 billion nutritional supplements every day. Do It Yourself (or DIY) Health as it is now called, is nothing short of the millennial phenomenon. The April, '98 issue of the Griffin Report, a food trade magazine, indicated that the sale of natural nutritional supplements (vitamins, minerals, herbs, amino acids, sports nutritional products, and diet aids) has grown 50% between 1992 an 1995, to a total sales figure of $6.3 billion, a figure expected to leap to $11.6 billion by the year 2000. It was also reported that in the past year the sale of herbal remedies alone increased by 48%, totaling $53 million.

With such large numbers of people taking natural medicines, it is clear that many want to prevent and enhance health in a natural way. I support this effort wholeheartedly, and am concerned that individuals make the correct decisions about which supplements to take. In most cases, people read about particular supplements and determine which ones they think would be good for them. In some cases, they visit a physician or nutritionist who makes certain suggestions. And, while this may help you make better choices, it is still a shotgun approach that neglects to consider your body chemistry, your constitution, and your lifestyle, in other words, the whole person.

For supplements to be most effective, they need to be tailored to your bio-individuality. Therefore, it is best if you are guided in your choices by using some type of system to determine your unique constitutional and/or chemical needs. As I've said in earlier chapters, there are several effective techniques with which a practitioner can test your tolerances and needs for individual substances. The Chinese Constitutional Types system I have presented in this book is one such method that can be very helpful.

Another strictly Western technique that uses a purely scientific method for determining bio-individuality is called TMA, or Trace Mineral Analysis. TMA measures your body's mineral levels to get a picture of your present chemistry. Sometimes referred to as hair analysis (because hair is the substance which is tested), TMA is, in my opinion, by far the most useful clinical tool for assessing which nutritional supplements a person needs at a particular time.

The process is simple, accessible, and very inexpensive. Approximately one tablespoon of hair (200-500 mg.) is taken (preferably from the nape of the neck). This sample is then sent off to a TMA laboratory where it is exposed to multiple acids and high temperatures which break down the hair, making the keratin (protein) contained in the third inner layer of the hair available for analysis. The minerals found in the keratin are then measured in quantities 1,000 times larger than the mineral concentrations measured in blood tests. The hair is analyzed using a highly sophisticated process called atomic absorption spectroscopy which measures its mineral concentrations. The minerals are measured in parts per million, and printed on a graph.

I've interpreted over 30,000 TMA samples over the years and have found them to be remarkably accurate, useful indicators of overall metabolic patterns in the body. Blood analysis, on the other hand, gives a poor reflection of the body's overall nutritional levels. This is partly because the blood is such a vital transportation highway, that the hypothalamus does everything it can to maintain the blood's biochemical equilibrium at all costs. In other words, all possible essential nutrients are directed first to the blood, and may be deficient in the rest of the body.

Hair (protein), on the other hand, is a much more accurate indicator of the true picture of one's biochemistry, and thus its biochemical needs. While I know that there has been some debate over the years about the efficacy of TMA, I feel very strongly that it is an excellent indicator of individual nutritional needs. However, it is crucial that a high–quality laboratory be used, along with an experienced practitioner who can correctly interpret the results.

## HAIR ANALYSIS CHART

### Elements Regarded As Toxic

| | | SAMPLE SIZE: | 0.15 g |
|---|---|---|---|
| | | SAMPLE TYPE: | head hair |
| | | DATE SAMPLED: | 01/01/1995 |
| | **HIGH** → | DATE IN: | 01/01/95 |
| | | DATE OUT: | 01/01/95 R |

| TOXIC ELEMENTS | PATIENT LEVEL (parts per million) | ONE STANDARD DEVIATION ABOVE MEAN | TWO STANDARD DEVIATIONS ABOVE MEAN → | MORE THAN TWO STANDARD DEVIATIONS ABOVE MEAN |
|---|---|---|---|---|
| Aluminum | 1 | ** | 8 | |
| Antimony | 0.100 | ********* | .15 | |
| Arsenic | 0.090 | ******** | .15 | |
| Beryllium | 0.010 | ***** | .03 | |
| Bismuth | <dl .001 | | .3 | |
| Cadmium | 0.300 | ************* | .25* | |
| Lead | 8.0 | *************4.5********* | | |
| Mercury | 2.90 | *************1.5********** | | |
| Nickel | 0.20 | **** | 0.7 | |
| Platinum | 0.001 | * | .02 | |
| Silver | 0.10 | **** | 0.4 | |
| Thallium | <dl .001 | | .05 | |
| Thorium | 0.002 | *** | ..01 | |
| Tin | 0.1 | ** | 0.8 | |
| Uranium | 0.280 | ************* | .2*** | |
| **TOTAL TOXIC REPRESENTATION** | ******************************************* | | | |

**Sample information**

OFFICE CODE: 2-2
ICP-MS analyzed
RACE: caucasian
HAIR COLOR: gray
HAIR PREPS:
SHAMPOO: glycerin soap

### Ratios

| | PATIENT RATIO | EXPECTED RANGE | |
|---|---|---|---|
| CA/MG | 18.7 | 5- | 15 |
| CA/P | 0.8 | 2.6- | 6.1 |
| MG/K | 0.1 | 1.8- | 5.0 |
| NA/K | 1.4 | 1.8- | 4.0 |
| ZN/CU | 13.9 | 4- | 12 |
| ZN/CD | 323 | >800 | |

### Elements Regarded As Nutrients

| NUTRIENT ELEMENT | PATIENT LEVEL (parts per million) | LOW ◆ BELOW 2 STD. DEV. | TWO STANDARD DEVIATIONS BELOW | ONE STANDARD DEVIATION (STD) BELOW | MEAN | ONE STANDARD DEVIATION (STD) ABOVE | TWO STANDARD DEVIATIONS ABOVE → | ABOVE 2 STD. DEV. ● HIGH | NUMERICAL VALUE OF REFERENCE RANGE ◆ ● |
|---|---|---|---|---|---|---|---|---|---|
| Calcium | 112 | ***************************** | | | | | | | 280- 600 |
| Magnesium | 6 | ***************************** | | | | | | | 30- 75 |
| Sodium | 109 | | | | | ********************* | | | 20- 90 |
| Potassium | 77 | | | | | ************************** | | | 9- 40 |
| Copper | 7 | | ********************* | | | | | | 11- 28 |
| Zinc | 97 | ************************** | | | | | | | 125- 155 |
| Iron | 8 | | | ********** | | | | | 5- 14 |
| Manganese | 0.16 | | ***************** | | | | | | 0.30- 0.75 |
| Chromium | 0.44 | | *********************** | | | | | | 0.80- 1.25 |
| Cobalt | <dl .001 | **************************** | | | | | | | 0.020- 0.045 |
| Vanadium | 0.010 | | | **************** | | | | | 0.009- 0.080 |
| Molybdenum | 0.070 | | | | | ********** | | | 0.030- 0.080 |
| Boron | 1.80 | | | | | ** | | | 0.80- 2.80 |
| Iodine | 0.1 | | ****************** | | | | | | 0.3- 1.2 |
| Lithium | 0.028 | | ******************* | | | | | | 0.050- 0.120 |
| Phosphorus | 134 | | *************** | | | | | | 144- 204 |
| Selenium | 0.290 | ************************ | | | | | | | 0.950- 1.700 |
| Strontium | 0.36 | | ***************** | | | | | | 0.50- 4.80 |
| Sulfur | 41000 | ************************ | | | | | | | 48000- 52500 |

### Other Elements

| ELEMENT | PATIENT LEVELS | EXPECTED RANGE | ONE STANDARD DEVIATION HIGH → | TWO STANDARD DEVIATIONS HIGH → |
|---|---|---|---|---|
| Barium | 0.21 | 0.40- 2.50 | | |
| Germanium | 0.008 | 0.003- 0.028 | | |
| Rubidium | <dl .001 | 0.020- 0.150 | | |
| Titanium | 0.440 | 0.100- 0.700*** | | |
| Zirconium | 0.300 | 0.020- 0.500*** | | |

COMMENTS:

When interpreting a hair analysis chart, even before I look at the nutrient mineral levels on the front page, I check the significant mineral ratios. (See the chart on next page).

In the lab format we use the first significant ratio CA/MG, which is calcium to magnesium has a norm of 7:1. The second ratio CA/P represents calcium to phosphorous which has a norm of 2.6:1. Third, we have MG/K, or magnesium to potassium which has a norm of 2.4:1. The fifth ratio is ZN/CD, or zinc to cadmium which has a norm of 800:1.

All of these are extremely significant markers of the metabolic chemistries in our bodies. For example, the second and third ratios, calcium and phosphorous and magnesium to potassium are both metabolic markers for the thyroid gland. They tell us whether or not the gland is operating at its most efficient energy level. The fourth ratio, sodium to potassium, reflects the energy output of the adrenal cortex—the outer layer of the adrenal gland. The ratio of calcium to potassium (not listed) is also an important factor in determining the metabolic functioning of the thyroid. If the ratio is either extremely high or low, it tells us that the thyroid is underactive. This is usually something that happens as a result of the sodium to magnesium ratio being extremely low. When sodium is very low in relation to magnesium, it indicates that the patient's stress levels are too high, the adaptability to stress has been very poor, and that emotional, mental or physical stress is overwhelming the body's chemistry and exhausting the adrenal medulla (the innermost portion of the adrenal gland). As I mentioned earlier, once the adrenal glands have become exhausted, they demand emergency support from the thyroid gland, which then becomes exhausted as well.

The fifth significant ratio, zinc to copper, is a very good indicator for progesterone and testosterone. The first, calcium to magnesium, is a good indicator for estrogens and androgens. Finally, the iron to copper ratio (not listed) also reflects the working of the adrenal cortex. So, the ratios of sodium to potassium, sodium to magnesium and iron to copper are primary adrenal markers. I look very carefully at these in relation to the ratios of calcium to phosphorous, magnesium to potassium, and calcium to potassium (thyroid indicators) because, once again, when the adrenal glands become exhausted, and the thyroid is pressed into service excessively, its ability to burn fat and others regulate the general metabolism is inhibited. This condition also decreases the body's ability to assimilate calcium. In many women with developing osteoporosis, the adrenal glands lie at the core of the problem. And simply putting such women on calcium supplements can create a host of additional problems. In most cases, the adrenal and thyroid glands need to be supported before the body can make safe and efficient use of the calcium supplements.

On the front page of the nutrient mineral analysis chart are the levels for 19 minerals, beginning with Ca, or calcium. The chart shows the normal reference range of each mineral as indicated by the pale, almost white horizontal (mean) strip in the center of the reference range. For example, calcium has a normal reference range of 280-600 ppm.; magnesium has a normal reference range of 30-75 ppm. etc. On the top of the nutrient mineral graph are the indicators for 15 toxic minerals. The levels for arsenic, beryllium, mercury, cadmium, lead, and aluminum etc. should in effect be zero, or as low as possible. Any indicators that these minerals are in the body is unfavorable and should be immediately addressed.

The following section contains a listing of the supplements and natural medicines that are most commonly indicated in the vast majority of TMA rest results I have interpreted.

**Vitamin A:** I use this for exceptionally low or high calcium levels as it is an excellent calcium balancer. In helping the body to assimilate calcium, it prevents excess quantities from depositing in the kidneys. I recommend that those with low calcium levels take 10,000 units of oil-based vitamin A along with 400 units of vitamin D every day.

**Vitamin B1:** I use this vitamin for exceptionally high or low adrenal ratio markers. (Extremely high or low sodium to magnesium, sodium to potassium, or iron to copper ratios tell me that the adrenal glands are working too hard or have exhausted themselves completely). In these cases I will recommend high doses of vitamin B1, also called thiamin, in a twice daily dosage of 100 mg with meals.

**Vitamin B2:** this vitamin lowers toxic mineral mercury and I also use it to lower elevated boron. High levels of mercury and/or boron indicate that the kidneys are inflamed and having a difficult time filtering proteins and cleansing themselves of endotoxins. When boron in particular is elevated, it indicates that vitamin B2 is deficient. In these cases I recommend high doses of B2: 100 mgs twice a day with meals.

**Vitamin B5:** Also known as pantothenic acid, vitamin B5 is needed whenever the ratios two, five and seven are displaced in a TMA chart. When the adrenal glands are overstressed, as indicated by these unbalanced ratios, I recommend 100 mgs of B5 twice a day with meals, for toning and strengthening. High sodium to potassium ratios also indicate to me that adrenal stress has exhausted the cardiovascular system. The higher that ratio goes, the great the cardiovascular stress. Vitamin B5 antagonizes sodium and potassium, taking the burden off of the adrenal glands and the cardiovascular system.

**Vitamin B6:** Also called pyridoxine hydrochloride, vitamin B6 antagonizes high copper levels which tend to build up in bile ducts, brain tissue, and liver tissue. This buildup tends to accompany inflammatory viruses and excessively high estrogen levels. They have also been linked to a myriad of health problems such as gall bladder disease, certain cancers in women, chronic retro viruses, and inflammatory disease such as rheumatoid arthritis. I recommend 100 mgs two times a day with meals.

**Vitamin C:** I like to use ascorbate (specifically vitamin C) to neutralize the effects of toxic minerals and endotoxins in the liver and kidneys. It is also a generally good immune enhancer due to its antioxidant properties. I recommend 3,000 mgs per day.

**Vitamin D:** I suggest vitamin D whenever calcium levels are extremely low. I specifically recommend doses of 400 units per day, along with Vitamin A to enhance calcium metabolism. (See vitamin A, above.)

**Vitamin E:** This vitamin works well in conjunction with vitamins B1 and B5 for adrenal support. Whenever ratios two, five, and seven are elevated or dramatically depleted, we know that the adrenal glands are working overtime and that they are stressing the cardiovascular system. Vitamin E is very good at lowering the excess stores of tissue sodium and potassium, taking the burden off the adrenal glands and the heart. I recommend taking 400 units per day of the d-alpha form of Vitamin E.

**Calcium:** I recommend calcium whenever I see that the TMA chart indicates extremely low calcium levels. I also sometimes recommend calcium when the chart shows extremely high calcium levels. This may sound contradictory, but often when calcium tissue levels are high, it indicates that calcium is not circulating in the blood, but is instead sedimenting (settling) into the tissues due to highly acidic blood. Calcium citrate will alkalize the blood and absorbs with great efficiency, rather than depositing itself as stones for example. Thus I prefer the calcium citrate form in a dose of 1000mg per day, taken in the same pill together with 500 mg of magnesium.

**Magnesium:** Along with calcium, magnesium is very important for alkalizing the blood and tissue, supporting the adrenal glands, and tranquilizing the nervous system when stress levels are high. Magnesium can also help with insomnia. (See recommendations for calcium above.)

**Zinc:** I prefer zinc gluconate taken in conjunction with vitamin B6 to lower elevated copper levels. I suggest a dosage of 50mg per day. (See also the section above on B6.)

**Iron:** When a mineral is low in the TMA, it usually indicates that the individual isn't able to assimilate the particular nutrient efficiently. Because of this, it isn't simply a matter of giving the nutrient, but also making sure that it can be assimilated. Iron bisglycinate is generally referred to as gentle iron because it is most easily assimilated and tends not to cause constipation. I recommend 30-50 mg of iron bisglycinate per day with meals.

**Chromium GTF** *(glucose tolerance factor)*: Low levels of chromium indicate to me that blood sugar is not being properly managed by the body, and it specifically suggest that insulin levels are either very high or low. This means that the patient most likely needs fewer high-starch carbohydrates, and should be eating more protein and low-starch carbohydrates. I recommend 200 mgs taken at mealtime once a day. If the chromium levels are lower than .01 mgs percent in the chart, I suggest taking two per day.

**Selenium:** Selenium is another very important indicator for thyroid. Whenever I see a TMA chart with extremely high calcium to potassium ratios and/or extremely high calcium to phosphorous ratios, I look right at the selenium because it reflects the activity of a thyroid hormone called T3, the most activating thyroid hormone. If I find low selenium, it suggests the likelihood of a low-thyroid condition. This situation is a good example of a case in which blood tests alone are particularly poor indicators of thyroid function. The best indicators are blood combined with TMA and basal temperature readings. (Underarm temperature should be 97.8)

**Multi-enzymes:** When I see elevated calcium, it indicates to me that calcium isn't being efficiently digested or assimilated, but is, instead, being stored in such places as the kidneys and arteries. Excess calcium can thus contribute to the formation of kidney stones and arterial blockages. Enzymes, specifically hydrochloric acid (available in multi-enzymes), are largely responsible for digesting calcium. Take one with each of three meals a day.

**Pectin:** I suggest pectin whenever I see elevated levels of mercury, lead, arsenic, beryllium, aluminum, or cadmium in the toxic mineral chart. Pectin binds with these toxic minerals to help carry them out of the body. Pectin should be taken in a dosage of two 250-mg tablets before bedtime so that it does not bind with other supplements or food nutrients.

**Raw Thyroid tablets and Raw Adrenal tablets:** These tablets are useful when imbalances are detected in the adrenal ratios (two, five and seven) in relation to the thyroid indicators (one and three). They contain ribonucleic acid which can bond with our cellular codes so that bovine sources from which they are made will actually strengthen the corresponding human organs. Once available only by injection in European health spas, these bio-regulating supplements are now available in freeze-dried tablet form. I recommend taking 150-200 mg tablets of raw thyroid and raw adrenal (from bovine sources fed on organic foods) with meals twice a day.

**L-tyrosine:** This amino acid is a direct precursor of both adrenal and thyroid hormones and its use is indicated when I see imbalances in ratios one, three and five. It helps control depression, anxiety, and appetite. I recommend 500 mgs taken twice a day between meals.

**Ciwugia:** Also known as Wild Siberian Ginseng, research has shown that ciwugia increases stamina and supports adrenal and thyroid function. I recommend using two 400mg tablets in the morning and afternoon on an empty stomach.

# CHAPTER 17

# The Spirit Ill at Ease

*How is your spirit ill at ease?*

*What is troubling you?*

*What are the patterns at work in your life
and how did they begin?*

These are the first and most important questions I ask of every patient I see. Regardless of your physical condition, I know that in order to heal, you must be whole, and that to be whole, your mind, body and heart must be integrated and nurtured. If you are not integrated, if you disregard your inner "spirit self," you will become disassociated, fragmented, and cut off from the animating source of your being.

I believe that the disintegration I see in so many people has come about as a result of our culture's focus on the external world. Where our ancestors once lived a more integrated spiritual existence, today's culture has become insensitive to the divine nature of the human spirit. Our materialistic bias has become our foremost mind-shaper, and popular culture has convinced us that we are little more than personality-driven bodies. The message in all this is clear: we are somehow incomplete if we fail to conform to the ideal materialistic image of who we should be. We have been conditioned by one pervasive message our whole lives — we are not good enough as we are; we must attain something outside ourselves in order to be complete. But the fact is that who we are does not depend upon what we have. Nor does ignoring any of the elements of self — be it mind, body, or spirit — help us achieve a peaceful, healthy, stress-free way of life.

The ancient Chinese believed that, at the subtlest level, our spirits 'ingest' everything we see, hear, smell, think, taste, and feel, and that we are fed and shaped by these influences. If, then, we bombard our senses with an endless barrage of sex, violence, and greed, if we burden our biological systems with toxins and intolerable foods, do we not become unhealthy in every sense of the word? And, since the truth is that we are spiritual beings, the conflict between the materialism we practice, and the needs of the spirit to be fulfilled creates chaos within us. I believe it results in disintegration, a sense of separation from the people around us, self-contempt, and ultimately . . . dis-ease. And we must become aware that, as our subtle spirits are traumatized by disintegration, we are creating bodily disease.

In one recent national survey, pollsters asked people if they were happy with their lives. Of the more than 50,000 respondents, only 18% said 'yes.' Thirty years ago, the same poll was taken and nearly 79% of respondents answered 'yes' to the same question. The question, of course, is 'why?' When I look into the hearts and minds of so many of those with whom I work each day, I see a growing mistrust in the world's social systems, its governmental authorities, and its institutions. Where we once perceived strength and integrity, we now often assume there to be only weakness, cupidity, and falsehood. We are in a socio-cultural phase of external disintegration, typified by the breakdown of social institutions such as marriage and family, and the onset of cynicism, fear, and uncertainty. In the process there is also disintegration between races, genders, and age groups.

The only way to begin to reverse the process is with the individual. Regardless of the present patterns in the external world, we must fulfill our human instinct to be integrated. There was a time when we could almost always count on the love, trust and integral support of the external world — mother, father, family, society. This is no longer necessarily so. Thus we must adapt to our circumstances and turn inward for the support, trust, and love necessary to to thrive and prosper. If it truly takes a village to raise a child, then we must create that village within ourselves.

Every Chinese Taoist was taught both fishing and farming. When there was no wind to propel their sailboats, they ate from their vegetable gardens. When the gardens were damaged by drought or flood, they set sail to harvest fish from the sea. In other words, they adapted themselves to fit the circumstances of their lives, and did so in a way that promoted harmony within themselves. We must also learn the art of adaptation between the universal poles of Yin and Yang, mind and body, spirit and ego. Now is the time to find our integration, our healing, and our wholeness within ourselves, to cultivate our own 'healing spirit.' The best way to do this is to integrate all the parts: the right brain with the left; our past with our present; our intuition with our logic; our emotions with our intellect; our vulnerable 'child' self with our powerful 'parent' self. In this way do we become truly aware of these polarities in our being, and learn to honor each of them.

As we work toward self integration, we will come to reclaim a sacred wholeness that holds the key to our healing. I believe that we all deserve to be whole, we deserve to heal, and we deserve to completed in love. But we must first acknowledge that completed love can only be engaged within an unconditional, autonomous, integrated human being.

The following is a script for a guided visualization that is aimed at helping you to integrate mind and heart. Please make a tape of it for yourself and listen to it frequently. I've used this program to help literally thousands of people cultivate a spirit of self-integration. It begins with a brief relaxation exercise. For best results, wear comfortable, loose-fitting clothing and find a time when you will not be disturbed as you do the exercise.

### INTEGRATION VISUALIZATION

*Relax. Take a slow, deep breath through the nose as you fill your lungs. Hold the breath, then release through the mouth. Once again, take a slow, deep breath through the nose, hold the breath, and release it through the mouth. Now, finally, take a third deep breath through the nose, hold, then release through the mouth.*

*As you relax, picture in your mind's eye your left foot and your left leg. Feel them both. Tense all the muscles in your left foot and your left leg; tighten them as much as you can. Now, take a deep breath through the nose as you continue to tense the left leg and foot. Now, at the count of three, simultaneously release both the breath and the tension you are holding in the muscles. One... two... three... now completely release the breath and the tension.*

*Next, focus your mind's eye and your attention on the right foot and the right leg. Tense all the muscles in your right foot and right leg as tightly as you can. Hold and intensify that tension for a moment. (Pause) Now, at the count of three, release the breath and release the tension and stress in the right foot and right leg. One... two... three... release the breath and the tension.*

*Now, focus your mind's eye and your attention on your left arm and hand. Tense all the muscles in your left arm and hand as tightly as you can. Hold and intensify that tension for a moment. (Pause)*

*Now, at the count of three, release the breath and release the tension and stress in the left arm and hand. One... two... three... release the breath and the tension.*

*Next, focus your mind's eye and your attention on the right hand and arm. Tense all the muscles in your right hand and arm as tightly as you can. Hold and intensify that tension for a moment. (Pause) Now, at the count of three, release the breath and release the tension and stress in the right hand and arm. One... two... three... release the breath and the tension.*

*Now, picture in your mind's eye your mid-torso, your stomach, your abdomen, your lower back, your upper back. Tense your abdominal muscles, your back muscles, your pectoral (chest) muscles, and as you do this you are preparing to sweep all the stress from all of these muscles and vital organs simultaneously with the release of the breath. But first, tense all of them up, then take a deep breath through the nose, hold that breath, tense the body even more, then, at the count of three, release the breath and the tension. One... two... three... release all breath and tension.*

*Now, in your mind's eye, picture your face, the top of your head, the sides and back of your head. Tighten up all of your facial muscles now. In a moment you are going to release all of the stress from your mind and from your thoughts. Take a deep breath in through the nose. (Pause) At the count of three, release all of your stresses and tensions as you breathe out through your mouth. One... two... three... release all breath and tension.*

*At this point, you feel very deeply relaxed. You are very aware of your entire being. You are in a deep, deep state of tranquil peace and relaxation. And now, as you rest peacefully, imagine that you are floating up toward a soft, puffy cloud. (Pause) You are traveling light as a feather, ascending slowly to that cloud. (Pause) As you reach the cloud, you settle yourself into it, lying restfully on that soft, comfortable surface. The cloud is your transportation through time. It will carry you back into the past, to a time in your childhood. Relax as you travel.*

*At last you slowly arrive at your destination. And, as you do, it's time to very slowly put your feet and legs over the edge of the cloud and let yourself float slowly down to Earth, still as light as a feather. You notice familiar surroundings and familiar faces. Perhaps you see your home, your neighborhood, your street. You see friends and family. As you continue to look around, you touch down at last and see your child self. He or she is whatever image you first picture in your mind. Regardless of whether or not your childhood memories are positive or negative, you are completely secure in your present state and you are happy to have this reunion with the spirit of your child self. As you see, feel, and emanate from your heart, your senses are drawn first to your child's natural innocence, which radiates from his or her eyes and heart.*

*Slowly, you approach your child self with all your natural instincts of love and nurturance. The world you left behind only temporarily blinded you to these instincts to love and nurture unconditionally. Now, as you gaze into the eyes of you child self, your deep desire to forgive, to love, and to nurture unconditionally are welling up from deep within you. Take this time now to speak from the heart to your child self. Send your thoughts, communicate your love telepathically.*

*Take some moments to enjoy this reunion. (Pause) Bask in this unification between your present and your past, your peaceful mind and your loving heart, your power and your vulnerability. Hold your child self close to you as your open your hearts to each other. Both of you are sharing in this long-awaited moment of tenderness. (Pause)*

*Now, ask your child self to come into your heart, to spiritually meld with you. Integrate this child deep within yourself. Tell your child, "I want to love and care for you, nurture you, and take you back with me so that you can become one with me unconditionally." (Pause) Then, slowly, let the spirit of your forgotten child self come into your heart. (Pause) You are rescuing that child from long suffering and an endless wait for your attention and love. You are now giving your child self a long-awaited, loving home in your heart. (Pause) This marks the end of your dis-integrated life, and the beginning of your integration. Feel the blending of your past with your present, your heart with your mind, your vulnerability with your strength. (Pause)*

*Together, you and your child self will rise up to the cloud that transported you here. Light as a feather, fully integrated, you both rise slowly to the top of the cloud. You rest atop the cloud, fully integrated and at peace. You body, mind, and spirit are one. You are filled with an internal sense of compassion and an unconditional love such as you've never known before.*

*You are transported back through time and space, once again arriving in the present. As your cloud arrives and gently stops, you sit up and dangle your feet over the edge of the fluffy surface. Lightly you float back to Earth, back into your daily life. But you enter your life as never before. Now all the care, all the love, all the support you've ever needed in your life is suddenly right there inside you, coming from deep within your own spirit. You know that from this time forward, you will always seek within yourself to fulfill your vital needs. You are no longer blind to the world's lie, and you are no longer victim to the world's false promise. You are fully integrated within.*

*Take a few minutes now to slowly return to the present moment. Do not rush off. It is important to reflect on what you have just done, and, most importantly, the person you are becoming.*

I have always found this integration visualization exercise to have a profound healing impact. Maximum healing begins with whole-ism and true human whole-ism is rooted in the solidarity of the mind, heart, and spirit at peace within a happy 'body home.' In my work, I often use the metaphor that refers to the mind as the father, the heart as the mother, and the spirit as the child. They all live together within the home (body), and only when the father (mind) and the mother (heart) are truly married to each other, is the child (spirit) safe to thrive and grow within a healthy home (body) environment. So, we can see clearly through this metaphor, that the physical health we all seek so desperately truly begins with autonomous integral self-hood. Practice the visualization above and I think you will be able to cultivate love and trust within yourself. In the process you will reintroduce your inner 'family' to each other. The closer together the parts of your 'whole' become, the closer you will be to knowing true and profound healing.

# Questions and Answers

**How can I lose weight safely and naturally, and keep it off?**

Eat three servings of fresh, whole, raw fruit, (not fruit juices) and three servings of fresh, whole, low starch vegetables daily such as; asparagus, broccoli, cauliflower, celery, green beans, kale, spinach, and summer squash per day. Also eat no more than two servings of starch such as; cereal, rice, pasta, potatoes, breads, and crackers. You must limit fat intake (oil) to two tbsp. per day and butter to two tsp. per day.

**Are there any natural food supplements that would naturally suppress my appetite?**

The amino acid L-Phenylalanine 500 mg., one mid-morning and one mid-afternoon. Also Psyllium Husk Powder, one teaspoon before meals three times daily in 10 oz. of water.

**Are there any food supplements that would naturally suppress my sugar cravings?**

The Amino acid L-Glutamine, 500 mg. one mid-morning, one mid-afternoon and the mineral Chromium GTF (glucose tolerance factor) 200 mcg. twice a day with food.

**Which snack foods are both healthy and satisfying?**

Almond nut butter spread when blended with rice syrup, dairy free soy cream cheese, and sugar free jams are all good tips for natural snacking.  Occasionally you can use a rice cream dairy free ice cream product as well.

**Can hair analysis in any way help me in my strategies to lose weight?**

Yes, hair analysis can help you better strategize for weight loss as it displays your mineral ratios of calcium to potassium which indicates how efficiently, or inefficiently, your thyroid is burning calories. Furthermore, by supplementing the amino acid L-Tyrosine, 1000 mg. a day on an empty stomach, you can help to rebalance your errant metabolism as indicated by this hair analysis ratio.

**Why are many over the counter weight loss drugs potentially harmful for me?**

Weight loss drugs not only artificially stimulate weight loss mechanisms in the body, but the heart and nervous systems as well. Thus they tend to elevate heart rate and blood pressure. In the long-term they can exhaust an already depleted metabolism further limiting the body's potential for weight loss.

## What is the best general form of exercise?

Research tells us that a minimum of thirty minutes of brisk walking three times a week lowers virtually all health risk factors while optimizing energy metabolism and weight loss potential.

## How can unmanaged chronic stress speed up my aging process?

The acid that builds up in your blood from chronic stress exhausts energy reserves at a far greater rate. In addition, the more stress hormones you secrete, the more you speed up cell death.

## How does stress cause heart disease and cancer?

Stress increases the body's productions of Glandular Hormones, which expedite the cellular loss of electrons. Once healthy cells lose their electrons, the probability of contracting cancer or heart disease is significantly increased.

## How does unmanaged stress affect my appetite?

Long-term stress increases the acidity of the body, which uses up vital nutrients more rapidly, thus increasing the appetite.

## What can I eat during periods of stress to reduce both my appetite and my stress levels?

Increasing your intake of raw fruits and vegetables during periods of acute stress will help alkalize your blood. This will reduce your appetite and stress levels.

### How can hair mineral analysis help me in my strategies for fighting stress?

The protein in your hair (keratin) is the best vehicle for determining the three key stress mineral ratios. These three are: sodium to potassium; sodium to magnesium; and iron to copper. These ratios are the keys to how your cells, vital organs and glands are capable of managing stress. Hair mineral analysis further gives clues as to how you can best support your body with diet and natural supplements during the recovery process.

### When my body nutrients are out of balance, am I more susceptible to the ravages of stress?

Yes. However, employing preventive means such as hair mineral analysis, proper diet and nutritional supplementation can significantly increase your adaptation response to stress.

### What is the best natural way I can reduce stress quickly?

Recent research suggests that the herb Kava Kava root is an extremely effective, safe and over-the-counter way to reduce stress quickly. Most studies seem to indicate that the average adult requires a dose of KavaKava root that provides a least 125 mg. of the root's active ingredient, Kavalactones, in order to be effective. I recommend 125-150 mg. of Kava Kava root along with a series of deep breathing exercises. Kava Kava should not be taken with any prescriptive pharmaceutical medications.

### What foods will improve my energy?

Increasing your intake of high starch carbohydrates such as whole cereal grains, brown rice, whole grain breads and pastas as well as potatoes, sweet potatoes, winter squash and fruits will generally improve your energy as they readily convert into glucose, the body's high octane fuel.

## Are there any safe natural supplements that will improve my energy?

The best safe energy enhancers that I know are a Twin Labs amino acid product called Glutamine Fuel or, Wild Siberian Ginseng. I recommend 500-1000 mg. of Glutamine Fuel or 500-1000 mg. of Wild Siberian Ginseng capsules taken daily. Both are best absorbed on an empty stomach, and should not be taken with prescriptive drugs.

## How can hair mineral analysis help me to increase my energy?

The hair mineral analysis ratio of calcium to magnesium is an important indicator as to how efficiently your glands and organs are processing glucose, the body's fuel for energy. If calcium and magnesium tissue stores are in balance and chromium and other mineral levels are low, you can increase your energy levels with 200 mcgs. of Chromium GTF (glucose tolerance factor) twice per day with meals.

## What can I do to relax my mind, and conserve energy in the face of acute stress?

500 mg. magnesium chelate per day will generally relax the nervous system. In addition, 50 mg. of 5HTP (hydroxy tryptophan) which is an amino acid can be used. It can be taken two times daily on an empty stomach. This will increase the brain's neuro-transmitters that relax and refresh the mind and body.

## Is there a natural way to improve sex drive and performance?

The hair mineral analysis ratio between zinc and copper is a vital hormonal marker that can reveal underlying sex drive and performance problems. When a problem exists there is often a high copper to zinc ratio. Thus 50 mg. of Zinc Gluconate along with 200 mg. of vitamin B6 and 800 IU of d-alpha tocopherol E will in time improve these conditions.

## Can you suggest an optimum sample menu for an average day?

*Breakfast:* two soft boiled eggs (soft-boiled eggs destroy their own cholesterol). For other protein options you may use a cup of sautéed tofu, 8 oz. of 1% plain yogurt, or 4 oz. of low fat cottage cheese. These proteins may be accompanied by either two slices of sourdough toast or a cup fruit.

*Lunch:* 4oz. of low fat protein: chicken, turkey, fish, tofu, or beans, with 10-12oz. of low starch vegetables such as broccoli, green beans, zucchini, and 1 cup of starch: brown rice, potato, whole grain pasta, or two slices of whole grain sour dough bread.

*Dinner:* repeat the same format as lunch, but vary your food choices.

NOTE: *Consult with your physician before taking any natural food supplements.*

Join our growing
MaXimum Healing Family

*Visit our web site @* MAXHEALING.com
*or call us at* 1–800–NBC–4545

# INDEX

# NOTES

## ABOUT THE AUTHOR

Mark Dana Mincolla, Ph.D., is a dedicated whole health counselor who has worked with more than 50,000 patients over 17 years as a nutrition and holistic therapist. He has captured his experience and knowledge in three books: Maximum Health, Your East-West Guide to Natural Health; The Tao of Ch'i: Healing the Unseen Lifeforce, and The Wu Way, a Path to Natural Healing.

Mincolla is known to audiences in New England through his Emmy-nominated weekly television segment on alternative health, Visions. He also has appeared on a number of nationally syndicated radio and television programs around the country. Mincolla's latest book, Maximum Healing is the subject of a national infomercial campaign.

Mincolla graduated from Franklin Pierce College with a B.A. in Psychology. He received an M.A. in nutrition from Goddard College and a Ph.D. in Health and Human Services from Columbia Pacific University. He has also studied directly with recognized Chinese masters of Eastern medicine and healing.